Praise for
The Jennifer Nicole Lee Fun, Fit Foodie Cookbook

"As the leader of culinary executions within this premier South Beach Destination, I understand the necessity of being well informed and organized in order to follow through with your original intent. JNL's book does just this by providing thorough information regarding recipes, ingredients, timeframes, and nutrition facts, and everything else you will need to truly convert to a healthier lifestyle.

Being in the business of food and family within the hustle and bustle of health-centric South Beach, information and variety are key ingredients for success. JNL's Fun, Fit Foodie Cookbook *provides access from all angles for people to be successful with leading a healthier lifestyle."*
—KELLY SHEEHAN, Executive Chef at Maxine's Bistro & Bar at the Catalina Hotel & Beach Club

"JNL is shaking up the healthy food industry just as I have shaken up the restaurant scene for over 18 years. Being an accomplished restaurateur and owner of two buzzing mega restaurants, I know firsthand just how important recipes, meal planning, depth in taste and the entire whole gourmet food experience is. JNL's Fun, Fit Foodie brand is doing this and much more, while keeping everyone's taste buds happy and waistlines fit and trim!"
—MICHAEL ARNETTE, Celebrity Restaurateur and Owner of Haven and Valencia in Atlanta, Ga

"Coming from a multicultural background myself, JNL's Fun, Fit Foodie Cookbook *has something in it that reaches all cultures. Plus the meals are incredibly delicious and fun to make! This is truly a must have book for all families and all health conscious people who still want to enjoy their food, that's full of flavor!"*
—CLAUDE TAYLOR, Director of Operations JNL WORLDWIDE INC., www.JNLWorldwide.com

"The Fun, Fit Foodie Cookbook *is a treasure chest of culinary and fitness inspiration. Jennifer Nicole Lee generously shares her mouth watering and innovative recipes, sought after nutrition knowledge and motivation in the pages of her recent book. As a busy mom and marathon runner, I will be enjoying JNL's* Fun, Fit Foodie Cookbook *in and out of the kitchen!"*
—CHARMAINE BROUGHTON-DUNN, Food Writer & Founder of MarathonMom.ca

"Having travelled the world, eating exotic meals, and meeting many beautifully fit women, all with their own special diets, I am glad to see that someone finally created a balanced food plan that all can enjoy. Cheers to Jennifer Nicole Lee and her fellow Fun, Fit Foodies!"
—MIKE BROCHU, Top Travel, Beauty & Fashion Photographer, www.MikeBrochu.com

Published by Advantage, Charleston, South Carolina.
Member of Advantage Media Group.

ADVANTAGE is a registered trademark and the Advantage colophon is a trademark of Advantage Media Group, Inc.

Printed in China.

ISBN: 978-1-59932-224-7
LCCN: 2011942505

This publication is designed to provide accurate and authoritative information in regard to the subject matter covered. It is sold with the understanding that the publisher is not engaged in rendering legal, accounting, or other professional services. If legal advice or other expert assistance is required, the services of a competent professional person should be sought.

Most Advantage Media Group titles are available at special quantity discounts for bulk purchases for sales promotions, premiums, fundraising, and educational use. Special versions or book excerpts can also be created to fit specific needs.

For more information, please write: Special Markets, Advantage Media Group, P.O. Box 272, Charleston, SC 29402 or call 1.866.775.1696.

Visit us online at advantagefamily.com

Fun, Fit Foodie™ is a trademark of Jennifer Nicole Lee. Other product names mentioned in this book enjoy specific trademark protections reserved by their owners.

The Jennifer Nicole Lee Fun Fit Foodie Cookbook

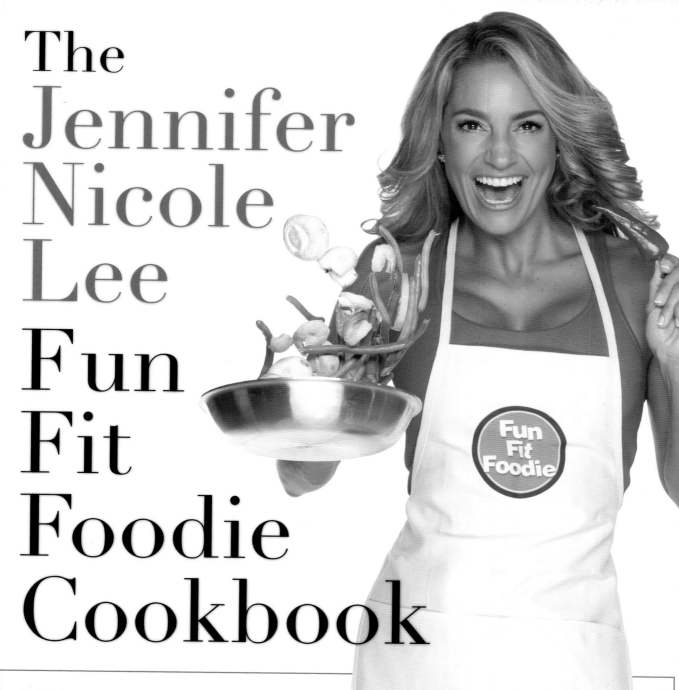

JNL'S SECRET SUPER
FITNESS MODEL™ **FAT BLASTING**
& **MUSCLE FUELING** RECIPES

Advantage®

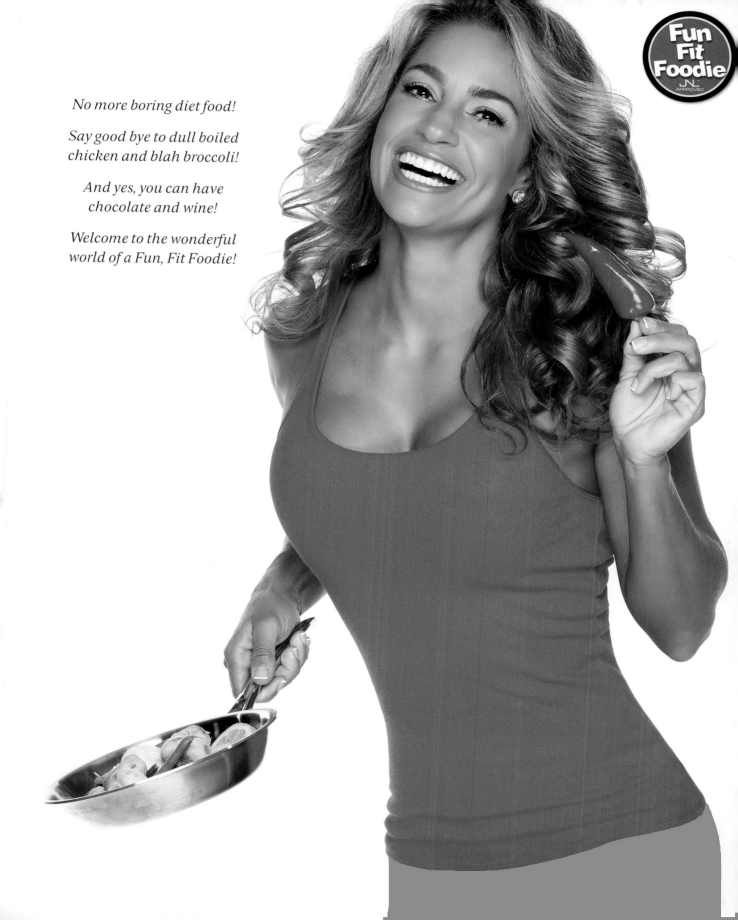

No more boring diet food!

Say good bye to dull boiled chicken and blah broccoli!

And yes, you can have chocolate and wine!

Welcome to the wonderful world of a Fun, Fit Foodie!

Fun
Fit
Foodie
JNL APPROVED

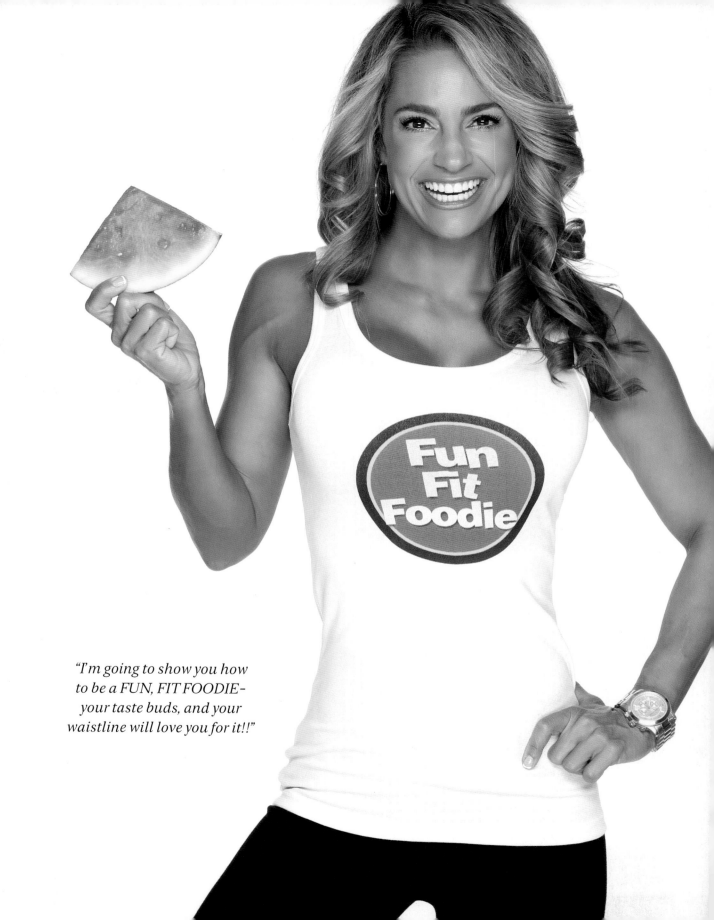

"I'm going to show you how to be a FUN, FIT FOODIE- your taste buds, and your waistline will love you for it!!"

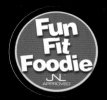

FOR MORE HEALTHY LIFESTYLE PROGRAMS, BOOKS, PRODUCTS, AND MATERIALS BY JENNIFER NICOLE LEE, PLEASE VISIT:

www.**JenniferNicoleLee**.com

www.**ShopJNL**.com

www.**JNLClothing**.com

www.**TheFunFitFoodie**.tv

www.**TheFunFitFoodie**.com

www.**JNLYouTube**.com

www.**JenniferNicoleLeeFB**.com

www.**FitnessModelProgram**.com

www.**GlutesThatSalute**.com

www.**JNLFusion**.com

www.**BikiniModelProgram**.com

www.**TheSexyBodyDiet**.com

www.**MindBodyandSoulDiet**.com

www.**JNLBooks**.com

DEDICATIONS:

This book is dedicated to all of my millions of JNL fitness friends, fans and "Fun, Fit Foodies" around the world - and to YOU reading this right now. It's my gift to those who suffered like me, trying to be healthy by eating boring diet food, or consuming little to nothing, and over-exercising. There IS a better way, and this is it. Cheers to all of you, and may you increase the quality of your lifestyle with this cookbook.

I believe in you!

–JNL

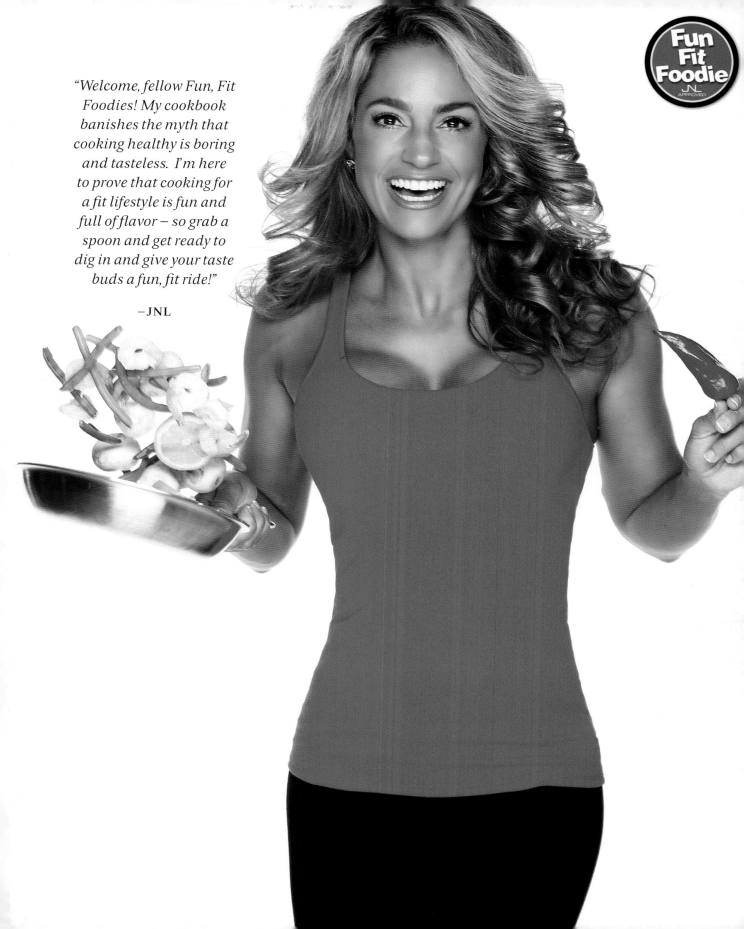

"Welcome, fellow Fun, Fit Foodies! My cookbook banishes the myth that cooking healthy is boring and tasteless. I'm here to prove that cooking for a fit lifestyle is fun and full of flavor – so grab a spoon and get ready to dig in and give your taste buds a fun, fit ride!"

–JNL

Fun
Fit
Foodie
APPROVED

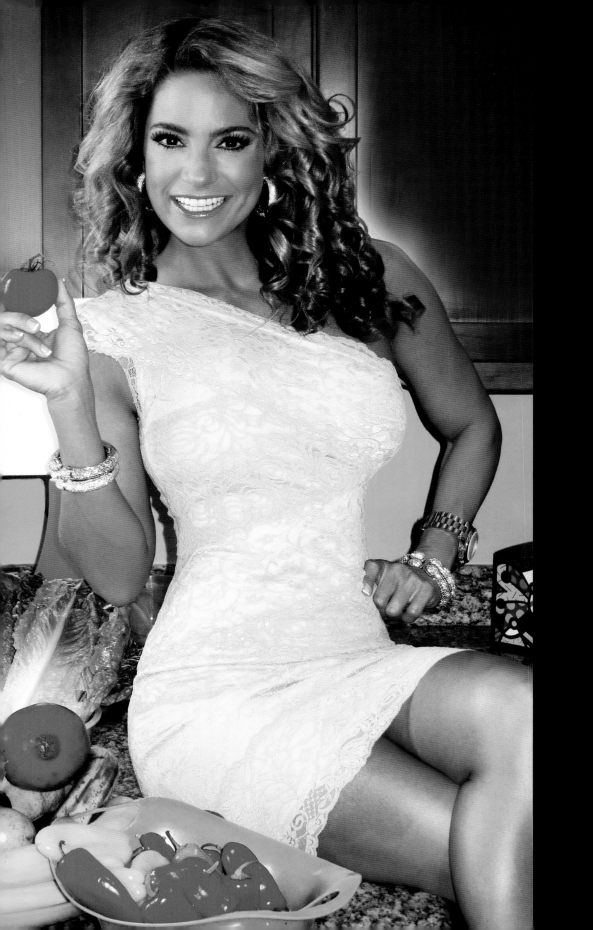

First of all, I'd like to thank God for all of my blessings, and giving me the desire to help others to improve the quality of their lives. Helping others achieve their healthy lifestyle goals is my life's purpose, and I thank God for giving me the inextinguishable passion, inner strength, desire and determination to achieve what I have thus far, and to keep me focused and motivated for the rest of my life's journey.

What truly makes me successful and joyful is my awesome family! I am so blessed to have the most amazing husband and soul mate, Edward Lee. Eddie, I have to thank you for being so dedicated and devoted as a loving, supportive husband and father. And thank you for eating all of the meals that I prepare for you!

The most awe-inspiring experience any woman can have is that of being a mom. I am so blessed to have the most amazing children. Jaden and Dylan are my everything! I thank you both for being the best two sons a mom could ever have! You are the best "taste-testers" and are brutally honest, making me a better cook. You teach me daily what true love is, and really what the important things in life are all about. I love you unconditionally! To my mom, Teodolinda Diodato Siciliano, a true Italian women who loved me through food! You taught me how to cook without ever using a recipe. As a little girl, I loved watching you in the kitchen where you usually worked most of the day to prepare and cook delicious meals that all of your four children loved. You are a true angel on earth.

To my dad, Rudolpho Girardo Siciliano, and to all the meals you ever prepared! I remember every Sunday growing up, how you would feed us all day long, with at least 8 courses that started in the early afternoon all the way until the evening. This tradition brought us closer as a family- and I was always intrigued how you never used a recipe, and just created super delicious dishes from whatever you seemed to find in your garden, pantry and 'fridge. You taught me to see endless creative possibilities with cooking.

To the best sisters I could ever have – Rosalinda and Valerie. Cheers to every meal we ate together growing up, and to the future meals we will have together. Both of you are beautiful from the inside out, and I am honored to be your sister. And thank you to my niece Gia and nephews Justin and Jared! Auntie JNL loves you!

To my brother, Johnny, who also loves to cook! For passing on the Siciliano name and cooking with passion.

Thanks to my book team for your endless hours of consulting with me, editing my manuscripts, and helping to pull the best out of me as an author and cookbook creator. Cheers to you!

Thanks to Advantage TV for producing such a high quality Fun, Fit Foodie TV Show. The time we spent creating the Fun, Fit Foodie TV Shows made memories that I will always cherish.

To all the JNL Fusion athletes around the world! Congrats to you all, for embracing such a powerful method of training and working out to the max. You all are workout warriors who expect the best and want the ultimate in a workout method. Thank you for spreading the word of the best workout to date, JNL FUSION!

To Debra Murray & Celebrity World Renowned, Chef Wolfgang Puck, for inviting me on live TV on HSN, allowing me to share my passion for cooking!

To My Coach and Celebrity Trainer, William Del Sol, for being my ever-reliable and super focused Coach! For your endless hours training and coaching me to be my fittest best. And for being on Team JNL FUSION. You ROCK!

To Unni Green, for your sweet spirit, positive energy, and always being so loving and kind. I applaud you for being an example of a Fun, Fit Foodie and super fit mom. And a big thanks for being a proud pioneer of JNL FUSION. Hats off to you!

To the beautiful, super-helpful and thoughtful women in my life, Neyda Purcachi, Claudia Gonzalez & Josepha.

To Tara, for being a real life angel on earth. And to your gorgeous daughter, Princessa Skye. Skye, you are such a blessing to all-with your sweet spirit and gorgeous aura. May God continue to bless you both.

To my best friend, Marli Resende, who is the most exceptional woman in the world. You are the strongest women I have ever met, and my nearest and dearest best friend for life. Your undying support and friendship is priceless to me. May God continue to bless you with prosperity, joy, wealth, health and abundance. I love and appreciate you!

"Indulging in one of my Fun, Fit Foodie™ meals gives me the same rush and enjoyment that I get when I finish one of my super-charged workouts in the gym. My body feels so good, from the inside out."

—JNL

"Learning to cook fit is not a one-time event, but rather a journey to be enjoyed...Celebrate fun, fit cooking by experimenting with a unique seasoning, tasting an exotic fruit, or trying out a rare vegetable!"

—JNL

To Zan and Mia, for being the best brother and sister Jaden and Dylan could have! And for also gladly eating the Fun, Fit Foodie meals I fix for our family time dinners. A family who breaks bread together, sticks together. I appreciate you both, as you are so loving and kind to Jaden and Dylan, and are outstanding people in my life.

Mike Brochu, who is the most brilliant and dedicated super-genius photographer in the world! Our Fun, Fit Foodie photo shoots in Miami, South Beach and New York City are priceless memories to me.

Thank you to Claude Taylor, aka "Mr Big" for being the best Director of Operations any company could have! I'm grateful for your fearless focus, your drive, integrity, fortitude, and relentless hard work ethic. I'm blessed to have a leader like you on my side!

To the Test Kitchen, for helping me check my recipes, to ensure the most accurate possible results. Because it's true, I'm Italian and I rarely use a recipe.

To Whole Foods, for allowing us to shoot in their amazing locations.

To Trader Joe's for providing us with wonderful, healthful and delicious food options, helping to make our meals just that much more fit and fun.

To BSN, for making the world's best supplements, which a Fun, Fit Foodie can rely on.

To Campbell's Soups, for helping us all to be a little more heart-healthy.

And to all of my super loving, loyal, positive, beautiful, and strong JNL Fitness friends and fans from around the world. Your emails, letters of support, phone calls, and reaching out to me show me that what I am doing is making huge improvements in the quality of your lives. I appreciate each and every one of you! I am grateful for all of you!

And lastly, thank you to the "Fun, Fit Foodie" in you! Having the desire to live a fit lifestyle without living in a constant state of sacrifice is so rewarding. I believe in YOU!

Cheers,
JNL

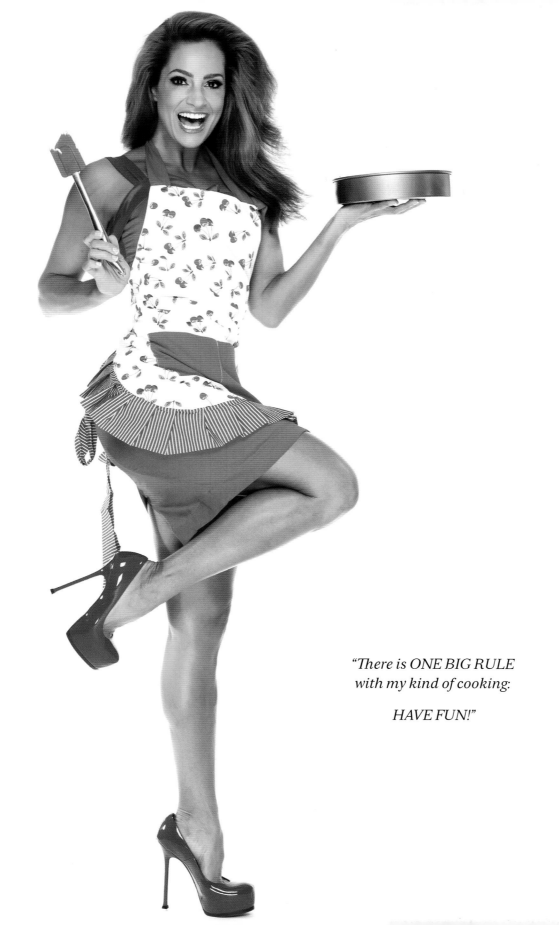

*"There is ONE BIG RULE
with my kind of cooking:*

HAVE FUN!"

"I guarantee that you will fall back in love with cooking healthy again, that you will enjoy these fresh, fabulous recipes that are great for your body and energy, and that your entire family will love them, too."

–JNL

CONTENTS

FOREWORD BY UNNI GREENE		17
LETTER FROM THE FUN, FIT FOODIE TEST KITCHEN		19
WELCOME		21
CHAPTER 1:	MY LOVE AFFAIR WITH FOOD!	22
CHAPTER 2:	HOW I DID IT	26
CHAPTER 3:	WHAT IS A FUN, FIT FOODIE?	32
CHAPTER 4:	HOW TO COOK LIKE A FUN, FIT FOODIE	40
CHAPTER 5:	THE FFF KITCHEN	48
CHAPTER 6:	BREAKFAST	54
CHAPTER 7:	LUNCH	66
CHAPTER 8:	DINNER & ENTRÉES	78
CHAPTER 9:	SOUPS & STEWS	90
CHAPTER 10:	SALADS	104
CHAPTER 11:	SIDES, STARTERS & HEALTHY SNACKS	112
CHAPTER 12:	DESSERTS	124
CHAPTER 13:	HOLIDAY FEASTS	134
CHAPTER 14:	TEA	142
CHAPTER 15:	WINE	146
CHAPTER 16:	FFF GUIDE TO EATING OUT & FAST FOOD	150
CHAPTER 17:	FAQS FROM FELLOW FUN, FIT FOODIES	154
CHAPTER 18:	FAT BLASTING & MUSCLE TONING WORKOUT GUIDE	158
BONUS:	THE 7-DAY JUMP START MEAL PLAN	162
ABOUT THE AUTHOR		169

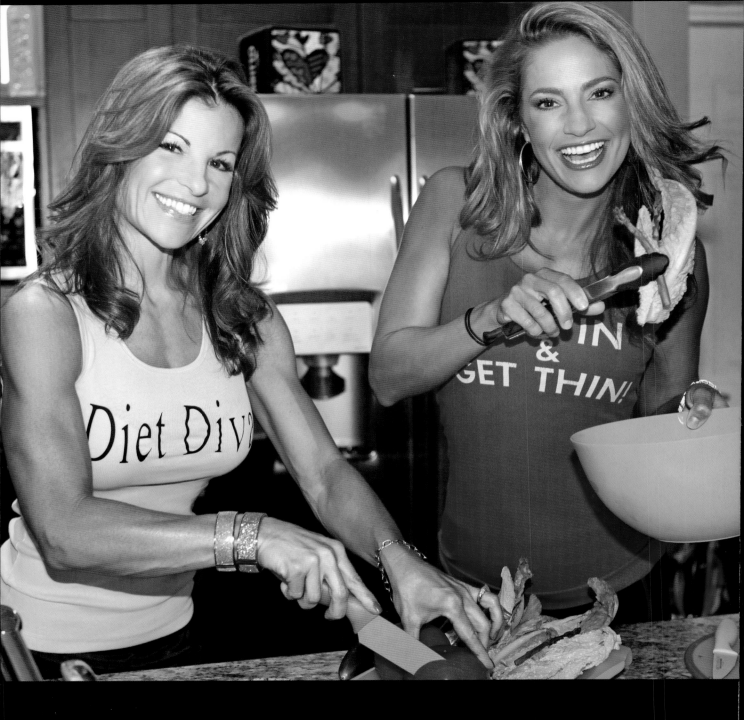

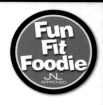

> *"You don't have to be a top gourmet chef to enjoy cooking and eating. I am a foodie who loves to live a healthy, fit lifestyle. This book will show you how to celebrate cooking fit for yourself and your loved ones!"*
>
> **–JNL**

◄ *Food Lovers & Fitness Fanatics and Friends, Unni Greene a.k.a. "The Diet Diva" and JNL in "The Fitness Model Factory" Kitchen*

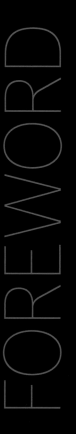

FOREWORD

Foreword by Unni Greene

The Fun, Fit Foodie. What a perfect name for a book that shows us yet another side of Jennifer than what we would expect, from one of the world's leading super fitness models and health and fitness gurus. Jennifer loves food!!!

We know that Jennifer has dedicated so much of herself to motivating others to get fit and healthy. She has already shown us what it takes, from the inside out, to commit to health and fitness. In her previous books, we learned what it takes from the mind, to get healthy and transform your life, as well as what it takes in terms of diet and exercise to get "super fitness model gorgeous." Now, she has blessed us with this fabulous, fun book that is a joy to read.

When Jennifer asked me to write the foreword, I was deeply honored. I have had the great blessing of being personally close to Jennifer and have been so enriched from watching her give her genuine love, concern and caring to others, as well as to myself. She is an incredibly unique woman, in that she is so gifted, physically, spiritually and mentally. I am in awe of her energy, zest for life and discipline. In this book, we get to see the fun loving, dedicated, real, every day wife and mother that Jennifer is. And we also get to learn exactly what it takes to embrace food instead of fearing it. To enjoy the flavors of unrefined, unprocessed, high quality foods without feeling guilty or putting on weight.

In this book, Jennifer shares her own personal struggles with weight gain and genetics. We learn how growing up in an Italian family, where everything centered around eating and food, became the source of her biggest challenge – her "fat gene." In this wonderful book, Jennifer teaches us how to achieve a lean, beautiful, healthy physique the "Fun, Fit Foodie Way." Incredibly enough, by eating this way, not only will you learn to enjoy food, but you will also stoke your metabolism to burn more fat and lose weight!

I love this book, because it encompasses everything you need to know about food and more!

This is not another diet book or a regular cook book at all. Instead, Jennifer gives us a lot of solid, scientific information presented in an easy to read, entertaining and interesting way. As always, Jennifer keeps her advice relevant and practical. You feel like you are right there with her as she tells you how to get the most out of your life. There is advice on how to stock your pantry and how to make sure you get your exercise. There are wonderful "Fun, Fit Foodie" Tips for you to enjoy throughout the book. Then, there are the recipes. They are all wonderful, flavorful and easy to prepare; super healthy, nutritious dishes that you can't wait to try. Each recipe is infused with Jennifer's personal story or touch! There is even a section on red wine and yes, chocolate! Both endorsed and enjoyed by Jennifer herself.

As the "Diet Diva," I know a lot about food and nutrition, but what Jennifer has put into this book is nothing short of amazing. As always, Jennifer makes me proud to be her friend and a student of all things that she so kindly shares. I know how thoroughly you will enjoy this book. It will soon be "dog eared" from all the times that you will pick it up and use it over and over again. Jennifer celebrates food, health and fitness and makes it fun and easy to do so.

All my love and eternal appreciation to the "Fun, Fit Foodie," my dear friend Jennifer Nicole Lee

–THE "DIET DIVA," UNNI GREENE

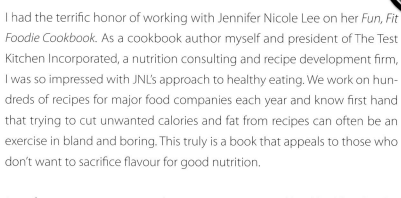

LETTER FROM THE FUN, FIT FOODIE TEST KITCHEN

I had the terrific honor of working with Jennifer Nicole Lee on her *Fun, Fit Foodie Cookbook*. As a cookbook author myself and president of The Test Kitchen Incorporated, a nutrition consulting and recipe development firm, I was so impressed with JNL's approach to healthy eating. We work on hundreds of recipes for major food companies each year and know first hand that trying to cut unwanted calories and fat from recipes can often be an exercise in bland and boring. This truly is a book that appeals to those who don't want to sacrifice flavour for good nutrition.

Jennifer wants you to succeed at your new, improved healthy lifestyle. She makes it personal by sharing her own experiences, her own pitfalls and her own successes. She puts her heart and soul into every page and her enthusiasm is contagious. And, once she's motivated you to make a change, Jennifer gives you the tools you need to achieve your goals.

This is not an elimination diet book; it is a book for people who live real lives. It is about embracing foods that are packed with nutrients and energy to make you feel good - body, mind and spirit. Jennifer knows, that without the occasional treat, life just isn't any fun, so this cookbook contains tips on how to indulge without compromising your goals. And, a healthy lifestyle involves more than just choosing the right foods. This book is also packed with motivational instruction on how to amp up your physical activity to boost your metabolism and burn off those excess calories. Jennifer has written this book with every type of cook in mind, and for those who are intimidated in the kitchen, there are plenty of tips on what equipment you'll need for culinary success, and even pantry stocking tips.

Our company employs a team of professional chefs, home economists and nutrition experts who are dedicated to the creation of delicious food. When I look at this cookbook, from a professional "foodie's" perspective, what I love are the bold flavours and the smart tips for replacing unnecessary fat, sugar and salt used throughout the recipe collection. Some of my personal favorites include:

- *Protein-Packed Sweet Potato Hash (on page 63):* A sweet and satisfying start to your day that will keep you from craving those high-fat breakfast pastries.

- *Indian-Style Beef Kabobs with "Snappy Bulgur" (on page 85):* Loaded with flavor and the healthy benefits of fiber.

- *Game Day Chili (on page 94):* Such a clever idea to use fiber-rich barley to add body and texture to this family classic without extra fat.

- *Apple & Walnut Endive Salad with Fresh Cranberry Dressing (on page 110):* Using cranberry juice concentrate to reduce the amount of oil needed in the vinaigrette is both genius and delicious.

And, of course, Jennifer has your busy lifestyle in mind by using time saving kitchen tools and techniques like a pressure cooker to shortcut meal preparation. Having worked with Jennifer and seen firsthand the passion and drive that she has put into these pages, I can't wait to see how you, her valued readers, take this book to heart.

BY AMY SNIDER-WHITSON
President, The Test Kitchen Incorporated, Professional Home Economist, Culinary Nutrition Consultant and fellow, Fun, Fit Foodie!

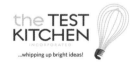

Protein-packed Sweet Potato Hash, page 63)

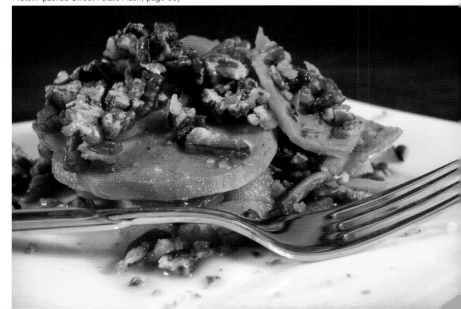

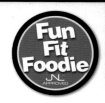

> "You CAN support your
> family and friends to
> be healthier, and live
> better, longer lives full of
> energy through the food
> you cook and serve to
> them. So enjoy being a
> Fun, Fit Foodie, not only
> for your health, but for
> your loved ones too."
>
> —JNL

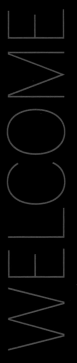

WELCOME

Dear Fun, Fit Foodie,

I love FOOD! And yes, food loves me too; I now have a healthy and balanced relationship with food. But it took me years to finally figure out that I deserve to eat healthy. Let's face it, there are a lot of other experts out there, but what sets me apart is that I am a true weight loss success story, who lost over 80 pounds after becoming a mom. I know what it feels like firsthand to be confused and frustrated about the conflicting expert advice in the nutrition and fitness world. But I sifted through all the fluff and developed my own tried and true methods of losing weight and cooking the Fun, Fit Foodie way. Don't get me wrong. This book is not a diet, or about eating food so flavorless that it's almost "sterile." It's about celebrating your inner cook. I wrote this book for all of you who are silently suffering from the big lie that your life has to be spent on an endless diet. I'm here to awaken your dormant love and passion for food, and of course to show you some cool, fun, easy ways you can bond with your family and friends over an amazing home-cooked and healthy meal.

I authored this incredible cookbook with you and your health in mind. As a leading fitness expert in the health and wellness field, I saw a serious need for a non-intimidating cookbook that would help others to learn to enjoy cooking in ways that would improve their lifestyles. Growing up, I only saw the extreme examples of cooking: the 250 lb. chef on TV who joked that "diet food" is what you eat while you wait for your steak and potatoes to finish cooking, or on the other side of the spectrum, the rail-thin "skinny-fat" fitness lady selling her idea of healthy eating, which was typically the "cabbage soup diet" or the orange and toast diet. There was no in-between. I am here to show you how to find the happy medium with my *Fun, Fit Foodie Cookbook*. This book is for those who love to eat, enjoy the "therapeutic" benefits of cooking and love to celebrate life with a great meal.

I'm proud to be a devoted mom and wife who finally realized that I could make my family healthier and happier by what I feed them. As women, we have the power to help those near and dear to our hearts enjoy longer, more vigorous lives, full of energy, stamina and zest.

This book is dedicated to all who know there is a more fun, more fit way of eating, and are ready to try it. Your body, mind, and soul will thank you! Cheers to all of you FUN, FIT FOODIES. —Jennifer Nicole Lee

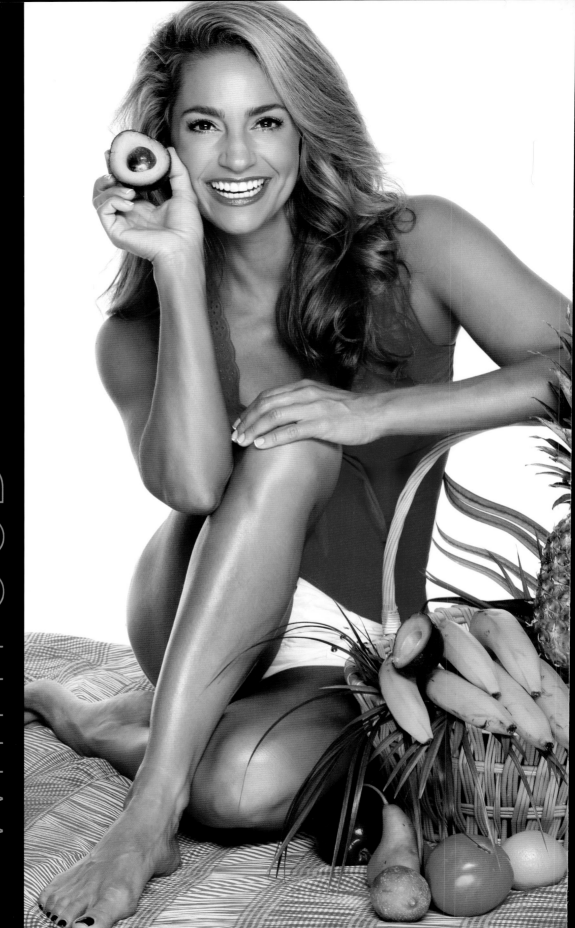

1. MY LOVE AFFAIR WITH FOOD

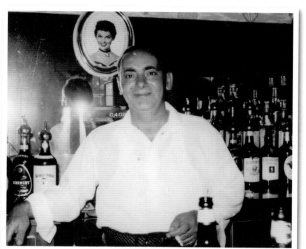

> *"Healthy food has always been the same old boring chicken and broccoli. In this book, I show you how you can enjoy 'good for you' gourmet meals that don't taste like cardboard!"*
>
> **– JNL**

How did I get into cooking? Actually, it all started with my passion for fitness, blended with my rollercoaster relationship with food. Being a first-generation Italian-American, it's practically a given that I learned about the importance of food, cooking and loving the "foodie" lifestyle very early on.

As many of you know, I lost over 80 pounds after the birth of my children, leading me to become a highly sought after fitness expert. The best part was that I did it by following my own food plans. I still had that "foodie" inside of me, even while I was losing the weight, and I was on a mission to find a way to combine the love of both fitness and food together.

Let me back up a bit. You see, my last name wasn't always Lee. My maiden name is Siciliano, and that's as Italian as you can get!

My mom was raised on the floor above an Italian seafood restaurant that was right on the ocean. She would peel shrimp in the morning. When I was born, and named after my grandfather Nicholas Diodato, he celebrated by cooking a big pot of homemade minestrone soup.

Funny — today, it's still one of my favorites!

My dad was born in Naples, Italy. My family was old-school Italian, and the biggest food lovers ever.

Growing up, every Sunday my sisters and brother would be bombarded by an all-you-can-eat food feast that lasted all day long. My dad would do all the cooking, and we would pretty much be at the table from about 11:00 in the morning to 8:00 at night, eating as many as eight different courses. The only breaks we would get from the table were to just get up and walk around a bit, or to help prepare the next course. Looking back at this weekly event, it's no wonder I was overweight as a kid. My job was the homemade pizza, which I loved to do, especially because of all the different meats we would put on the pizza. Sometimes I helped out with the lasagna. The greatest gift my parents gave me was the love for food that is still with me today.

Ultimately, it all caught up with me. I ended up yo-yoing on the scale, and the only weight loss method

My grandfather: Italian-born chef and restauranteur, Nicholas Diodato

I knew was the "starvation diet" of eating little to nothing, and exercising obsessively. I knew this could not be healthy, but I didn't know of any other way to "get fit."

Moving to Miami, with its cultural expansiveness, Cuban-infused foods, and Caribbean influence, my taste buds were in heaven! I'd never heard of taking pork fat, frying it, and eating it as a snack. Then, the beans and rice, and fried plantains? I mean come on! Unfortunately, my weight rocketed to the heavens, too.

I met my husband, who is Chinese/Jamaican, and I learned about an entirely new culture, gained some new great recipes, and, yep, a lot of new-found pounds (hang tight — I've got a killer Jamaican Red Pea Soup recipe in the Soups & Stews chapter!).

It was time to get real with myself after I had my children. I got in the best physical condition of my life, but still could not stick with the boring, bland diet food that many promoted. My love for food and fitness inspired me to create this book for you.

> *"I love watching The Food Network. Being a fitness expert, I would always watch the foodie shows, and ask myself 'How can I make this gourmet recipe healthier? How can I make it even more delicious, while making the recipe lighter?' This mind set helped me to become the Fun, Fit Foodie!"*
>
> **– JNL**

My Story of Yo-Yo Dieting, and My Love/ Hate Relationship with Food

"So what do you want to eat today?"

This food-focused question was the first thing I was asked when I woke up. Every morning, it was a serious topic of discussion over a fattening breakfast of fried eggs and sausage, prepared with love by Mom. Sometimes, discussions over what the day's menu would entail ended in a heated debate; my sister wanted lasagna while my brother wanted spaghetti with meatballs and sausage. Eating was an all-day affair with no breaks! And no matter what I said, it was coming my way, and large portions of it.

Clearly, my mom and dad showed their love for us through food. Well, what do you expect from an Italian family? The notion of food as a medium for love was passed down from generation to generation, and it was the only thing they knew how to do. I inherited the "fat gene." The correct medical term would be a slow metabolism. My slow metabolic rate further worsened because I was constantly presented with poor food choices and large portions. Growing up, I gained and stored weight so easily. Do you ever feel sometimes that all you have to do to gain 5 pounds is just look at a piece of chocolate cake? Well, that was me!

We were always eating. When we were happy, we would celebrate and eat. When we were sad, we would mourn and eat. When we were bored, we would eat to pass the time. And when we were planning a special occasion, we would build the event around a festive menu. It was always about food and what the next meal was.

When my parents separated, they ratcheted up the stakes by waging "food wars." My mom would constantly ask me, "So, whose lasagna is better, mine or your father's?" My dad would seem a little peeved if we went to his house on a full stomach from our mom's. He would ask, "So what did she feed you?" Both of them seemed to put a lot of energy into strategizing plans to "one up" each other on the next meal. You can see how I was brainwashed into believing that food was truly the end-all!

And, boy, did I yo-yo. When I got desperate to lose weight, I'd either not eat much, or simply not eat at all. My body horded the fat pounds instead of losing them. It is a crazy, but common, diet cycle that may have helped some of us temporarily lose weight, but in the end only makes us gain it all back, or even more, after our diet ends.

Have you ever felt like a gerbil, running on one of those stationary wheels, going nowhere fast? That's what the endless unhealthy cycle of losing and gaining feels like. With my Fun, Fit foodie lifestyle, your outcome will be different! As a Fun, Fit Foodie, the foods you eat combined in my tried and true recipes will help you to burn the fat while feeding the muscle, thus transforming your body into a fat burning machine, unlocking your fat-burning and weight-loss potential.

This food plan will help you to understand and overcome the core of the problem: your metabolic rate. In this miraculous book you'll find so many great recipes that you will be armed with a wide array of food choices and meal ideas you can use at any time. I like to call it having ammunition to fight fat with! I drastically changed all the associations I had been taught about food, into the positive tools I use in this book. In doing so, I was able to transform my body into a fat-burning machine, unlocking my weight-loss potential by stoking my metabolic rate.

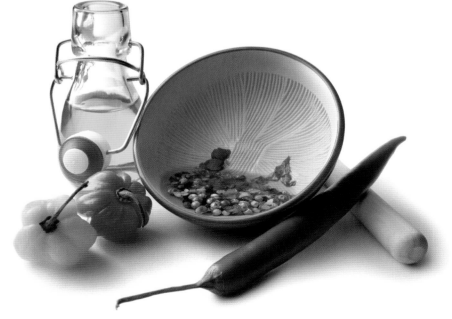

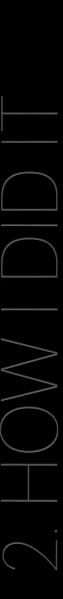

2. HOW I DID IT

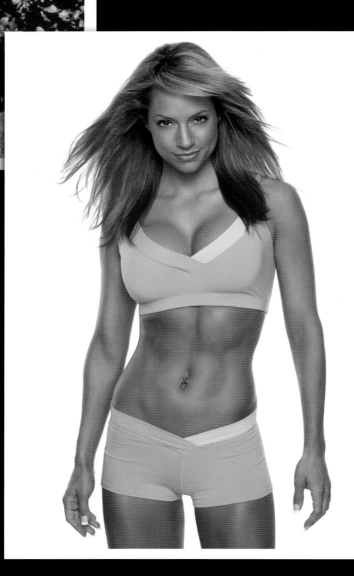

How I lost over 80 pounds as a Fun, Fit Foodie, kept the weight off and still enjoy my food!

The "Aha" Moment that Changed My Life

I t was an ordinary summer day, but a day that changed my life forever. I will never forget it. It was mid-May, official swimsuit season. And I had a friend brave enough to take a picture of me in a fuchsia bikini. I didn't know it at the time, but this was to become my famous "before" picture.

When my brave and willing friend handed me that photo, I couldn't believe my eyes. Was that me? What happened; where did I go? And who was that fat woman wearing my bathing suit? I literally did not recognize myself. I knew I had gotten out of shape, but good grief, did I really look that bad? I'd been fooling myself, masking my weight with baggy black clothes, lots of makeup, and big hair. But that day, I stripped my daily costume away and put on a bikini to get real.

And, boy, did I get real with myself! Talk about instant motivation. From that point on, I did all I could to lose the weight and get in shape. I placed that photograph in my bathroom so I could see it every day when I got ready in the morning. I saw it at night before I took my shower. There wasn't a day that I did not look at that photograph and say to myself, "You can do better; this is not who you were meant to be. Realize your potential and work hard at achieving it. You can do it! If not now, then never!"

This get-real moment was fueled by horror stories I'd heard from other moms I met at the park. One lady confided in me that ever since the birth of her baby, she had not been able to lose weight. I asked her how old her baby was and she responded, "Oh, my son is 5 years old now."

It was all I could do not to gasp out loud. How could this be? Five years passed with no weight loss? This could easily have been me, but that "before" picture and my "aha!" moment gave me the shove I needed to take my life in the right direction. I built my lifestyle around a sound food plan and exercise routine that I created in order to build lean muscle, melt off fat pounds and add energy to my life, enabling me to look and feel my best. It can do the same for you – all you have to do is get started.

> *"The only real stumbling block is fear of failure. In cooking you've got to have a what-the-hell attitude."*
>
> **—JULIA CHILD**

How Do You Start?

BEFORE YOU BECOME A FUN, FIT FOODIE— TAKE YOUR BEFORE PHOTO!

My advice is to take a "before" picture of yourself, look at it honestly, and ask, "What can be better? What would I like to change?" Remember, I went from being a miserable overweight mom to being crowned Ms. Bikini America. You can improve the way you feel and look with my Fun, Fit Foodie meals, just as I did.

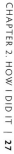

Yes, there are many health benefits to becoming a Fun, Fit Foodie and cooking like one. Given the new, healthy way of eating you'll learn, and the smarter food choices you'll be making by the time you've cooked your way through this book, you too will look and feel better. So, to document your success, grit your teeth, and take your BEFORE photo. And then, about three months into this Fun, Fit Foodie way of eating, take your "after!" I know you will be super-surprised at your own transformation, from the inside, out!

BE CREATIVE

What do I mean by "be creative"? I don't mean that you have to be an artist or a philosophical thinker. But we are in this for the long run. Being healthy is a process, a journey, not a one-time event. Fitness and health are going to be the basis of your new lifestyle. Therefore, we need to make it fun, full of variety, and interesting.

Being creative is one of the fundamental points of being a Fun, Fit Foodie. Ask yourself, "What are my favorite foods, and which are the sorts of exercise that I most enjoy?" If you answered "Italian food," then buy a low-fat, low-carb Italian cookbook and learn how to remake your old favorites. And, if you love to play tennis, join a tennis club or hire an instructor who will help you strengthen your backhand or give you a better edge on your game. If you love nachos, be creative and reinvent the recipe using low-fat ingredients, rather than the real stuff. Just open your mind to

> *Being creative is one of the fundamental points of being a Fun, Fit Foodie." Ask yourself, "What are my favorite foods, and which are the sorts of exercise that I most enjoy?"*

new and different approaches and add them to the bag of tricks that will help you fight the war on fat. By being creative, you will make it fun, refreshing and interesting. There will never be a dull moment in your new, healthy life.

PUT FITNESS FIRST, FROM THE KITCHEN TO YOUR GYM!

Well, not exactly first, but make it a top priority. It should be a rock in your life. Your kitchen should be a Fun, Fit Foodie sanctuary with healthy cheats and treats, ready when hunger strikes! And yes, LIFE will happen! So just plan ahead on sticking to your exercise routine, regardless of the challenges or changes life will throw at you.

If your car breaks down, calm down with exercise. If you get a job promotion, celebrate with exercise. If your husband leaves you, get over the guy with exercise. No matter what happens —stick to your routine! Of course we all will have bad days and fall off of our diets — but it's never the end of the world, unless you let it be. Refocus yourself, look at your compass, and get back on track.

And prepare to be tempted. This strategy of "thinking five steps ahead" will allow you to win at the game of fat loss. For instance, say that you know that you have to attend a family cookout. What should you do? Be a smart, Fun, Fit Foodie and execute your fitness plan: munch on a crispy apple before you go to the party. This will fill you up, cutting the edge off of any uncontrollable hunger pains that might set in while you are there. Then opt for the grilled chicken breast with no bun, a side salad, and an ear of corn with no butter. You've won by putting fitness first and you are still able to enjoy your family's social activities without sabotaging your fitness goals!

SET YOURSELF UP FOR SUCCESS

Put health on the shelf and the gym bag in the car! Everywhere you go and no matter where you are, your healthy habits will follow you! If you plan ahead and make following your routine as easy on you as possible, it will be almost impossible to not stick to your plans and reach your goals.

- Stock your fridge and pantry with the latest guilt-free snacks and Fun, Fit Foodie treats. Low-carb and low-fat foods taste better and are better. Try something new today.
- Have your gym bag ready to go in the car for a pre-or post-workday workout. Throw in a towel and a change of clothes, and you will have no excuse to skip the gym.
- Buy exercise DVDs (try my JNL FUSION exercise DVDs, your body will thank you!) and have them ready to go in your family room.
- Have your running shoes right by the bed so all you have to do is roll out of the sack and head straight to your home gym, or bang out a JNL FUSION DVD workout in your living room.

Why Being a Fun, Fit Foodie will Help You Be Healthier without Stress

You'll probably be surprised to learn that I don't count calories, I don't count fat grams, and I don't weigh my food. And during my weight loss transformation, during which I lost over 80 pounds, I didn't do any of those things either. In contrast, the only time I did count calories is when I was stuck in the loss/gain cycle, and yo-yoed up and down the scale. Every time I went that route and put myself on another dreaded diet, I would weigh my food, count my calories, and count my carbs. I knew how much sodium, sugar, and fat grams were in practically every bite! My attempt to school myself into healthy eating practices turned more into a dreaded science and math class. No fun at all! Eventually I would lose patience, lose count, and gain weight.

When I finally and forever gave up calorie counting, I stopped harassing myself and creating extra stress on me. For me, calorie counting just didn't work, and to this day I am still going strong – and without the extra headache of "math homework"!

I'm happy to say that most of my fellow Fun, Fit Foodies don't need to rely on counting carbs, or colored cards, or even points, to enjoy living a Fun, Fit Foodie lifestyle. What we do, as followers of the fast-growing fitness foodie trend, is enjoy our food. We relish our exotic flavors and bold spices. We celebrate our daring food combinations, and embrace a new-found freedom to eating healthy.

Ask any doctor, cardiologist, personal trainer or licensed nutritionist why some people burn off fat quicker than others. The unanimous answer is their metabolic rate. Metabolism can be defined as the rate at which we burn off calories. Our metabolic rate is, for better or worse, an inherited characteristic. But in this case, your DNA doesn't dictate your destiny, because this is where my *Fun, Fit Foodie* recipes come into play. The meals will help you to blast fat while feeding muscle. These recipes will work with your body to help you to increase your metabolic rate and lose weight.

increase your metabolic rate, right off the bat. It is this; you must increase your lean muscle mass. I'm not going to waste your time. It is simple math. To add muscle, you'll need to follow this tried-and true weight-loss success formula: weight train and then fuel the growing muscle with a proper, nutritious food plan that is based on moderate to high levels of protein, fiber-rich carbs, and good-for-you fats. Period.

There are no "diet cards," no "phases," no "steps" or "for two weeks do this, and for two weeks do that" stages. I'm going to keep it simple, short, and sweet. Good, solid, proven information, which will be transformed into power in your life, is what you will find in the Fun, Fit Foodie lifestyle

> *I will give you the necessary tools and steps that will actually stoke your metabolism, turning your body into a roaring furnace that burns off the fat even when your body is at rest.*

Lots of the latest fad diets instruct you to cut out fruit. Fruit in the *Fun, Fit Foodie* meal plans is a powerful super food, which is essential. How could a credible fitness expert tell you not to eat fruit for 2 weeks? How misleading! As a specialist in sports nutrition and a top VIP Celebrity Master Trainer, I would never ask you to do something so ridiculous, harmful, and unsafe.

I will give you the necessary tools and steps that will actually stoke your metabolism, turning your body into a roaring furnace that burns off the fat even when your body is at rest. These steps, in combination with healthy habits in general, will allow you to finally crack your weight loss code and unlock your weight loss and fat-burning potential.

In my simple plan, there are no band-aid approaches. I would like to introduce you to a proven way to

Of course if you don't eat sweets or have any alcohol the first two weeks of any diet, you will lose weight. That is not rocket science and you don't need to be a doctor to know that. But it's not necessary to make yourself miserable in order to lose weight. In the *Fun, Fit Foodie* food plan you will be shown not only how to get the number on the scale down, but to keep it down forever while you gain strength and ramp up the energy in your body. In addition, you'll be improving your appearance and overall health.

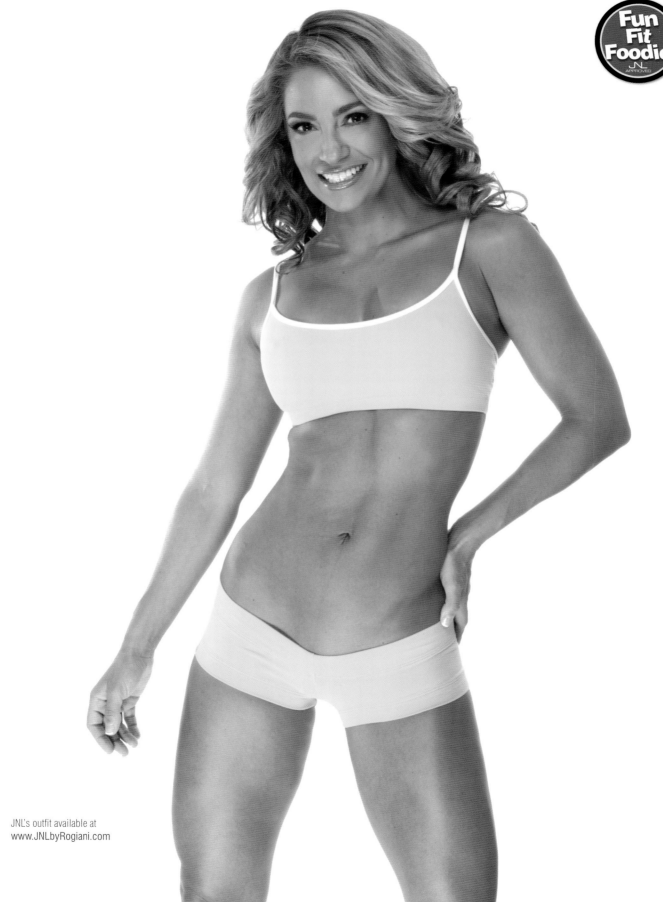

JNL's outfit available at
www.JNLbyRogiani.com

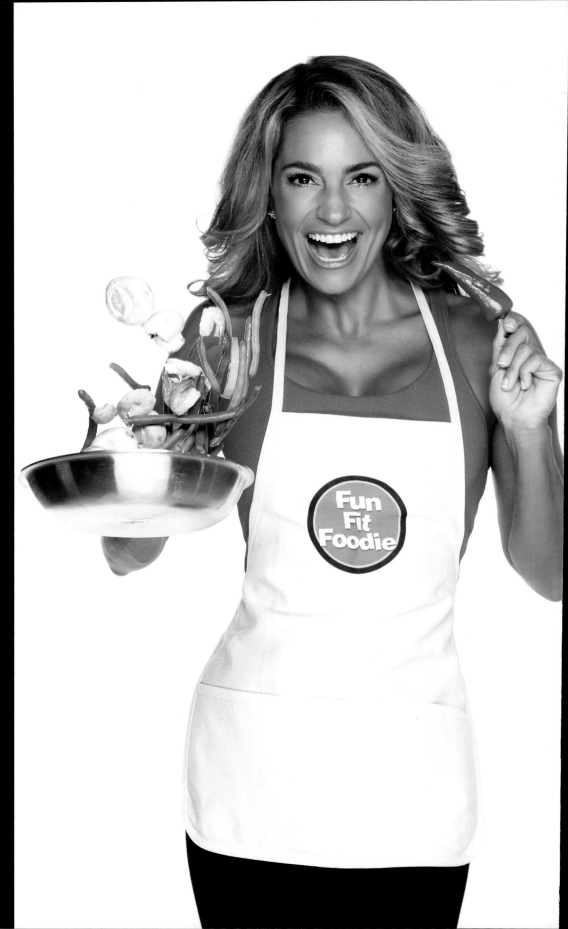

Let me explain
exactly what a
Fun, Fit Foodie is,
and what it is that
we stand for.

3. WHAT IS A FUN, FIT FOODIE?

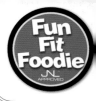

Fun, Fit Foodie Credo:

"I'm proud to be a Fun, Fit Foodie! The meals I choose and prepare help to increase the quality of my health. I am excited to learn new methods of cooking that will help me cut out unnecessary sodium, fat, calories, carbs, and sugar. I believe that it's fun to cook fit. I enjoy exploring new, fit recipes that are chock full of antioxidants, that are farm fresh or organic, and will help me to love the way my body looks and feels!"

THE 10 COMMANDMENTS OF THE FUN, FIT FOODIE!

1. I will avoid processed foods whenever possible.

2. I will choose organic or farm fresh foods when they're available.

3. I will choose wild fish, free-range chicken, and grass-fed, antibiotic-free beef whenever I can.

4. I will not rely on the salt shaker for seasoning my meals and use more sodium-free seasonings and fresh herbs instead.

5. I will limit cooking with butter and lard and switch to cooking with healthier fats like olive oil and coconut oil more often.

6. I will free myself from deep-fried foods, and choose instead to steam, poach or sauté foods using a heart-healthy oil such as canola oil.

7. I will reduce the use of refined sugar to sweeten my deserts or meals wherever possible, and use organic honey in its place.

8. I will include a range of different colored vegetables in each meal, in order to get as many antioxidants into my meals as I can to fight off free radicals.

9. I will enjoy the health benefits of tea by drinking one cup every other day, or more.

10. I will enjoy eating whole grains, such as barley, quinoa, brown rice, in place of white breads, white pastas and refined carbs.

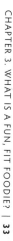

The Basic Fitness & Lifestyle Principles of the Fun, Fit Foodie!

Let's get to the core of the *Fun, Fit Foodie* principles so that we can stoke our metabolism, and start blasting the fat off before we know it. These basic principles will soon become part of your daily healthy lifestyle. The Ten Basic Principles to living a Fun, Fit Foodie lifestyle are:

- *Eat frequently!* Aim to eat 5 to 6 meals a day, including breakfast, lunch and dinner, and including two to three snacks. A Fun, Fit Foodie's eating plan looks like this; breakfast, snack, lunch, snack, then dinner, followed by an optional snack.

- *Eat smart!* Front load your calories in the morning and at lunch to get your metabolism working and fuel you appropriately for the day.

- *Have a tea party!* Drink green tea and see how it speeds up your metabolism.

- *Eat high protein foods* to promote satiety and prevent hunger cravings.

- *Enjoy an occasional indulgence*, including the "forbidden" anti-diet foods, such as wine and chocolate. Being a foodie means you get to enjoy chocolate, and also to salute with an occasional glass or two of red wine. Both chocolate and red wine have been proven in several studies to actually reduce your chances of the #1 silent killer of women, heart disease. Visit www.heart.org, the official website of the American Heart Association to find out more about cardiovascular health.

- *Exercise in the morning*, to work with your metabolism, and to fuel the "after-burn" so that you continue to burn calories more efficiently throughout the day.

- *Lift weights* and the fat will fall! The 3 F's that equal an A+ in weight training: Form, Focus, and Full Range of Motion!

- *Circuit Train*; JNL Fusion is my weight training and cardio circuit program. Visit www.JNLFusion.com for more information. Don't Hit a Plateau —Keep Your Body Guessing!

- *Train in your target heart rate* — not under or over!

- *Don't over-train.* Take time to rest.

EAT FREQUENTLY, EAT SMART

In my second book, *The Jennifer Nicole Lee Fitness Model Diet*, I explained the wise way to work in your calories throughout the day, and how to concentrate most of your calories at the beginning and the middle of the day. I cannot stress enough the importance of eating a hearty, healthy breakfast.

> *"Eat breakfast like a queen, lunch like a princess, and dinner like a peasant!"*
>
> —JNL

Breakfast is the most important meal of the day. It should also be your largest and most filling meal. Your metabolism will be more efficient when you front-load your calorie intake in the morning. You will eat less at night, helping you fight off those extra pounds that creep up from late-night eating. And your body will function more effectively when it's correctly fueled in the morning after your nightlong fast. That hearty breakfast will work with your body to get it fully charged and primed to burn fat. A good breakfast sets you up for successful eating, thwarting any mid-morning hunger pangs.

A weight-loss client of mine, Laura from Arizona, would argue that she was saving calories by not eating breakfast. I took a look at her food log and it told me what I had feared and expected. She was so ravenous by lunch that she would eat enough for three people! I showed her how cutting out breakfast actually caused her to over-eat and consequently make poor food choices for lunch because by lunchtime, her body was crying out for food. She wasn't a "breakfast person," but I convinced her that it was necessary to get into the habit of eating a balanced meal of protein, good-for-you carbs, and fats in the morning.

When she took my advice and made a healthy breakfast a regular part of her program, the results spoke for themselves. She had more energy in the morning, ate less at night and her hunger died down, allowing her to be in more control of her food choices throughout the day. She thanks me to this day for helping her retrain her eating habits to include the morning meal so that she could "trickle down" the calories throughout the day.

You'll want to:

- Aim to eat 5 to 6 times a day, 3 meals and two snacks. You need to reward yourself with a constant even flow of calories that will keep you fueled all day long.

- Aim to have a balance of protein and good-for-you carbs and fats in each meal or snack you consume.

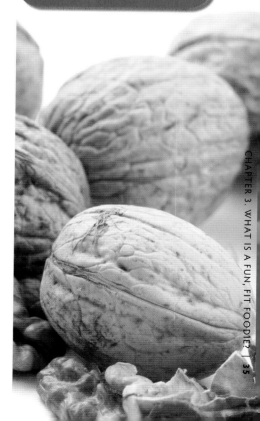

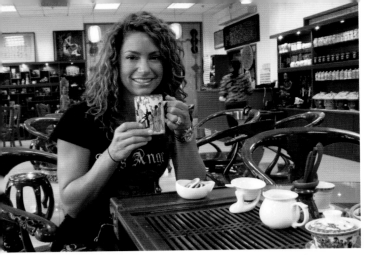

JNL visits an ancient tea house in Bejing, China

HAVE A TEA PARTY!

Although green tea has a moderate amount of caffeine in its chemical makeup, studies show that there is an interaction that occurs between its active ingredients that promotes increased metabolism and fat oxidation. Green tea extract has substantial implications for weight control, especially when taken during the daytime. A person taking green tea extract will increase his or her energy levels by 4% during a 24-hour period. Since thermogenesis (the rate at which the body is able to burn calories) contributes to about 8-10% of the daily energy expenditure in a typical person, this 4% increase due to green tea translates into a 35-43% increase in daytime thermogenesis.

In addition, green tea extract does not raise the heart rate and blood pressure nor does it over-stimulate your adrenal glands, as do many prescription weight-loss drugs. The best way to incorporate green tea into your weight loss/fitness regimen is to purchase a brand of organic green tea that contains 150-200 mg. of antioxidants. This tea can be purchased at most grocery and health food stores. Start by either taking green tea extract in a supplemental form, or by drinking a cup of tea every day. Plan to drink green tea with meals to increase your metabolism as you eat.

EXERCISE IN THE MORNING

Don't get me wrong, exercise at any time of the day is great. But to get the maximum potential out of any exercise routine it is absolutely essential that you do your EXERCISE IN THE MORNING!

I am living proof that anyone can retrain themselves to wake up earlier, and get in an early morning exercise session. I was never a morning person; I often slept in late and went to bed late. This late-to-bed and late-to-rise habit was in direct correlation with the way my body hoarded all that extra weight for so long! I'm here to tell you that I changed my sleep habits, and so can you. Some mornings will be hard, but you just have to stick to it. You can do it! If not now, then when? So, set your alarm at least 40 minutes earlier, get your workout clothes ready the night before, and decide what type of exercises you are going to do, so that there is no last-minute guesswork. Just jump out of bed, and begin jump-starting your metabolism. And believe me, you will start to enjoy waking up early in

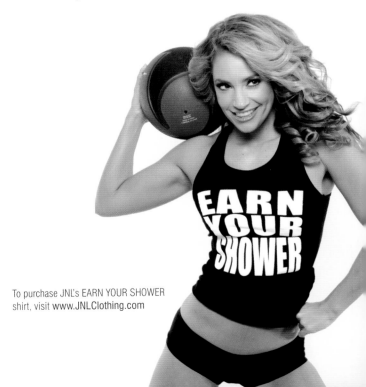

To purchase JNL's EARN YOUR SHOWER shirt, visit **www.JNLClothing.com**

the morning while everyone is still sleeping (this time will become your special time, devoted to you and just you). You will get hooked and actually look forward to that alarm going off in the morning, reminding you that it is time to give back to yourself with a rewarding dose of good, old-fashioned exercise.

Gyms open early especially for early birds, and even provide hot coffee and group exercise classes with a peppy instructor to get your engines revved for the day ahead! Here are the benefits of making the morning your choice time to exercise:

- Revs up your metabolism for the entire day.
- Helps set your biorhythm for the day.
- Helps you sleep better at night.
- Increases your energy level throughout the day, and rewards you with a better sense of self-control.
- The jump-start of morning exercise helps your body to continue to burn calories more efficiently throughout the rest of the day. Like exercising without even trying!
- Provides a better outlook on the day ahead.
- Makes you feel refreshed, alert, and ready for anything that may come your way after your morning exercise.

Some mornings, you may only be able to fit in a 10-minute walk, but it's important to try to do something every morning. Consistency is the cornerstone to success! If you train yourself to exercise first thing in the morning, it is more likely that you will stick with it over the years and build a foundation of success.

Exercise also helps control the appetite. Morning exercisers vouch that their appetites are suppressed or regulated for the day, and that they aren't as hungry. This allows them to make better food choices. Morning exercise works like a natural appetite suppressant, without having to take a pill. A number of people have also told me that it puts them in a "healthy mindset" that makes good eating choices easier to make throughout the day.

If you exercise at about the same time every morning, and ideally wake up at about the same time on a regular basis, your body's endocrine system and circadian rhythms adjust accordingly, and physiologically, some wonderful things happen: A couple of hours before you awaken, your body begins to prepare for waking and exercise because it "knows" it's about to happen.

It is also MUCH easier to wake up. When you wake up at different times every day, it confuses your body, which is never really "prepared" to awaken. Set your alarm clock so you wake up at the same time every morning, even on the weekends. This will train your body and mind to get your optimal rest at night and be your most productive during the day!

Your metabolism and all the hormones involved in activity and exercise begin to elevate while you're sleeping. You feel more alert, energized, and ready to exercise when you do wake up. Hormones prepare your body for exercise by regulating blood pressure, heart rate, and blood flow to the muscles.

Setting an appointed time every morning becomes something you will look forward to. You are doing something good for yourself by setting aside time to take care of your body and mind. Many find that it's a great time to think clearly, pray, plan their day, or just relax mentally. It is an all-in-one therapeutic session that is free, with multiple benefits.

Another great side effect of regular exercise is clearer thinking. Research has demonstrated that exercise increases mental acuity, and that this increase on average lasts 4 to 10 hours after exercise. No sense in wasting that while you're sleeping.

Another big plus to an early bird exercise routine is that the crowds typically found at the gym in the afternoon will be a non-issue for you. Exercising first thing in the morning is the only way to ensure that something else won't crowd exercise out of your schedule.

When your days get hectic, exercise usually takes a backseat. If finding time to exercise is difficult, you need to rethink your schedule, recognize exercise as a priority in your life, and plan to get up 30 to 60 minutes earlier to make the time for it. If necessary, try to go to sleep a little earlier. That shouldn't be difficult; in fact, research has demonstrated that people who exercise on a regular basis have a higher quality of sleep, and thus require less sleep.

MAINTAINING YOUR TARGET HEART RATE

It is very important that you maintain your target heart rate when you exercise. To receive the full benefits of exercise you need to pace yourself. When beginning an exercise regimen, it is important to find out what your initial target rate is so that you can determine your fitness level and track your progress.

Your target heart rate should stay between 50-85% of your maximum heart rate. If you do not have a heart rate monitor, you may use the "conversational" monitor:

- If you are able to hold a conversation and walk or exercise at the same time, you aren't working too hard.
- If you are able to sing, as you're exercising, you are most likely not working hard enough.
- If you get out of breath too quickly and have to stop to catch your breath, you are working too hard.

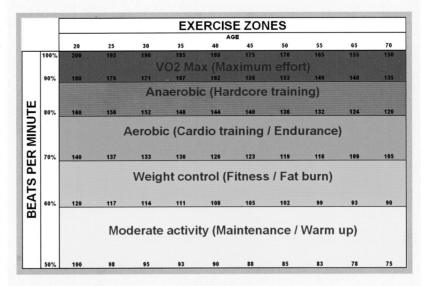

EXERCISE ZONES									
AGE									
20	25	30	35	40	45	50	55	65	70
100% 200	195	190	185	180	175	170	165	155	150
VO2 Max (Maximum effort)									
90% 180	176	171	167	162	158	153	149	140	135
Anaerobic (Hardcore training)									
80% 160	156	152	148	144	140	136	132	124	120
Aerobic (Cardio training / Endurance)									
70% 140	137	133	130	126	123	119	116	109	105
Weight control (Fitness / Fat burn)									
60% 120	117	114	111	108	105	102	99	93	90
Moderate activity (Maintenance / Warm up)									
50% 100	98	95	93	90	88	85	83	78	75

BEATS PER MINUTE

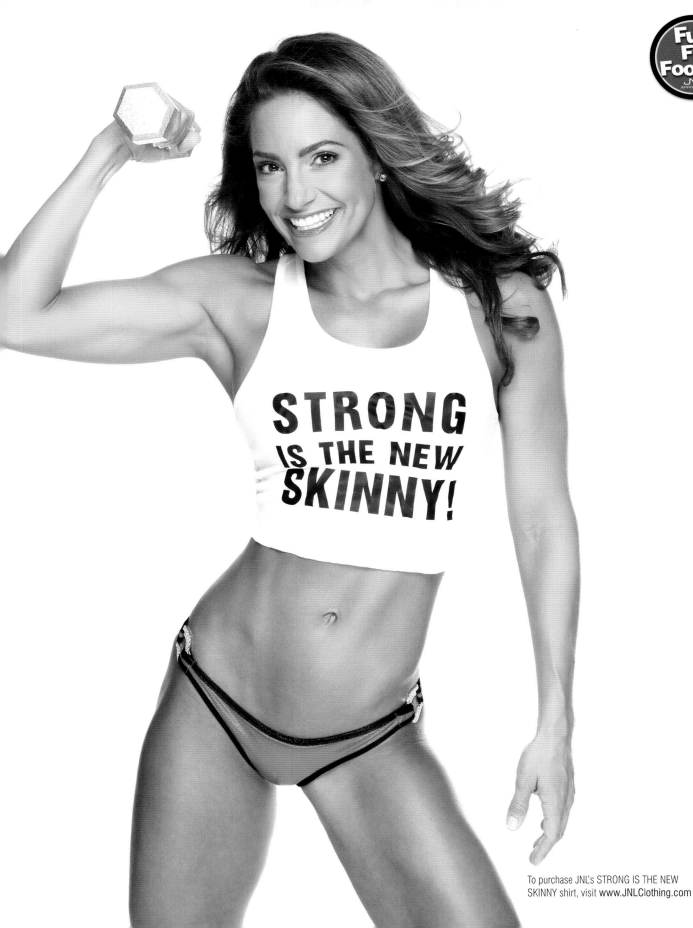

To purchase JNL's STRONG IS THE NEW
SKINNY shirt, visit www.JNLClothing.com

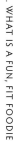

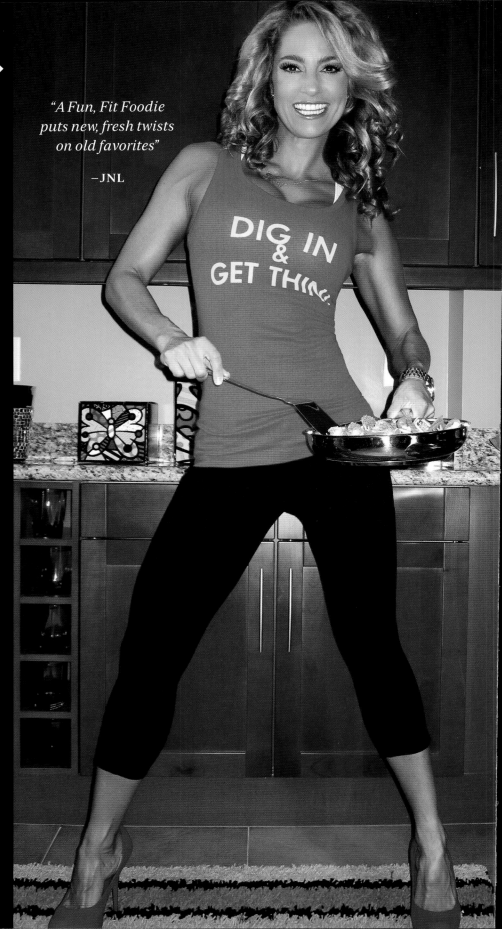

JNL in her colorful and fun "Fitness Model Factory Kitchen" ▶

"A Fun, Fit Foodie puts new, fresh twists on old favorites"

–JNL

4. HOW TO COOK LIKE A FUN, FIT FOODIE

Banish the Myths of Healthy Cooking

"We spend countless hours cooking, in front of the table eating, at the market shopping, and in our kitchen prepping and preparing food! Why not make it all worth our while and cook the Fun, Fit Foodie way?"

—JNL

> *"I'm proud to be a Concoction Queen in the kitchen! I'm known to take favorite recipes and meals and revamp them, taking out all the unnecessary fat, carbs, sugar, and calories, but leaving in all of the flavor!"*
>
> —JNL

> *"This is my invariable advice to people: Learn how to cook – try new recipes, learn from your mistakes, be fearless, and above all, have fun!"*
>
> —Julia Child,
> *My Life in France*

To purchase JNL's DIG IN & GET THIN shirt, visit **www.JNLClothing.com**

D o you need to get fitter, but still love to eat? Or do you think you are eating healthy, but just don't feel as good as you should? Running out of steam early in the day, and not sleeping well at night? Have you tried the starvation diets, to lose weight only to gain it back? Well, my Fun, Fit Foodie lifestyle plan will help solve all of these all-too-common problems. There are certain daily food rituals that Fun, Fit Foodies enjoy.

Myth:
Healthy food and cooking are boring with a capital "B."

Truth:
Healthy foods and healthy recipes are exciting, fun, and easy to prepare.

So what makes a *Fun, Fit Foodie* meal just ohh sooo memorable, yet superhealthy? Well, the super food ingredients, spices, and exotic flavors! And, of course, how you enjoy your foods throughout the day, starting with a breakfast that's the biggest meal of the day. Read on to find out more about the Fun, Fit Foodie way of celebrating eating!

Here are some of the basic "must do's" to be in the Fun, Fit Foodie group, and they are absolutely a joy to do, like:

- Use heart healthy oils in cooking and discover flavorful, versatile coconut oil.
- Incorporate lean protein sources throughout the day.
- Eat lots of fresh, unprocessed fruits and vegetables including full-fat avocado.
- Choose whole-grain and complex carbs.
- Low-sodium and salt-free seasoning to add flavors to meals.
- Use low sodium broth when making soups, stews and gravies.
- Always eat a big, healthy, metabolism-revving breakfast full of whole grains, lean proteins and fibrous carbs.
- Indulge in good for your heart red wine and dark chocolate.
- Munch on nuts and seeds.
- Drink green tea, white tea and herbal teas for calorie free thirst quenching.
- Create scrumptious tummy-filling soups and stew (made even easier by using your pressure cooker, just push one button!).

"One thing we all share as human beings is our passion and love for food!"

–JNL

"Cooking is a serious art form and a national sport."

–JULIA CHILD, My Life in Franc

So read on, and learn how to tease your taste buds while fulfilling your fitness and healthy lifestyle goals!

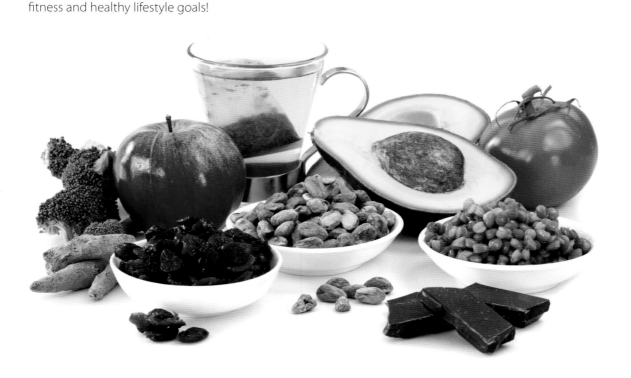

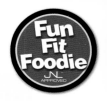

Sample Menus

FOR BREAKFAST:

- Egg white omelet with veggies and low-fat cheese with a side of whole wheat toast.
- Low-fat milk smoothie blended with protein powder mix and your choice of fruit (my favorites are strawberry-blueberry and banana peanut butter).
- Salmon, low-fat cream cheese on a small whole-wheat bagel.

BODY REWARDING MORNING SNACKS:

- Apple, with 2 tablespoons of peanut butter.
- Low-fat, low-sugar yogurt.
- Low-fat string cheese with a side of sliced tomatoes, drizzled with olive oil and salt-free Italian seasoning.
- Nutritional shake.

LUNCH:

- Grilled chicken salad with a small whole wheat roll or side of whole-wheat crackers.
- Blackened salmon with a side of steamed vegetables and brown rice.
- Tuna fish salad made with a touch of low-fat or fat-free mayonnaise, on a bed of fresh, crisp greens, side of whole-wheat crackers or whole-wheat roll.

BODY REWARDING AFTERNOON SNACKS:

- Handful of almonds (about 12 pieces) and a pear.
- Banana sliced lengthwise, smeared with 2 tablespoons peanut or almond butter, drizzled with honey and accompanied by a handful of wheat thins.
- Low fat cottage cheese with a dollop of sugar-free preserves.

DINNER:

- Baked tilapia with sweet potato and side salad.
- Seared Asian seasoned tuna, with a side of seaweed salad and miso soup.
- Grilled flank steak, sautéed tomatoes, and brown rice, small side salad.

Fun, Fit Foodie Heart Healthy Foods

HAVE YOU FED YOUR HEART TODAY?

I love my heart, and it "hearts" me back. And you too can show your ticker a little bit more TLC on a daily basis by following my *Fun, Fit Foodie Cookbook*. From sweet potatoes to asparagus, every bite of heart-healthy food gives your body a super-charged serving of phytonutrients. They repair and prevent damage to cells, thus preventing the #1 silent killer of women, heart disease.

We can also sip our way to a healthier heart. By toasting to your health with a bold cabernet sauvignon, you can reduce your risk of getting heart disease.

This recipe book is loaded with the Fun, Fit Foodie-approved heart-healthy foods listed below. Make sure you incorporate them into your meals, and make it a point to keep the more highly portable snack options ready to eat when hunger strikes. And, yes, your heart will thank you!

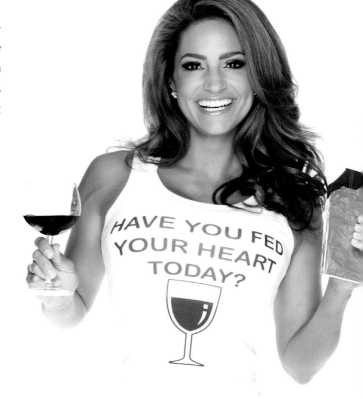

- Red wine
- Dark chocolate
- Tea
- Blueberries
- Brown rice
- Flaxseed (ground)
- Oatmeal
- Salmon
- Black or Kidney Beans
- Avocado
- Extra Virgin Olive Oil
- Olives
- Almonds

- Walnuts
- Tomatoes
- Acorn squash
- Spinach
- Broccoli
- Red bell peppers
- Asparagus
- Oranges
- Sweet potato
- Cantaloupe
- Carrots
- Papaya

> *Here's to a cheers and to a chunk!*
>
> – JNL

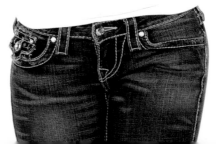

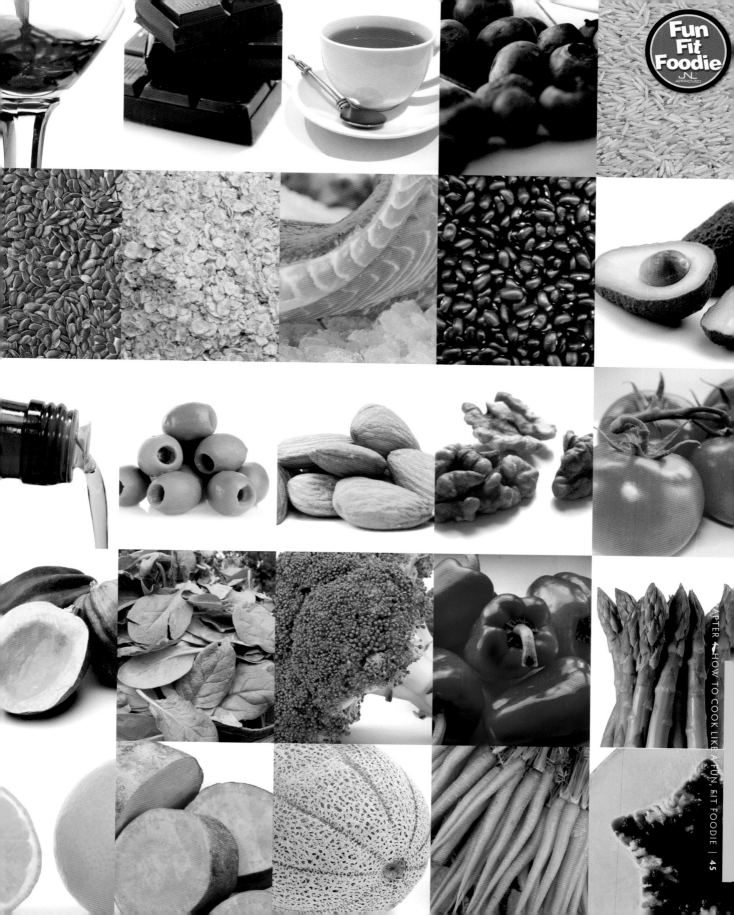

Fun, Fit Foodie's Fast Explanation of Oils

Oils, oils everywhere! Once it was all about fat-free eating, but now experts tell us that we actually need oils and fats (the right kinds, of course) to be our healthiest and best. Here is my rundown of what oils you need, and how to use them!

Fats and oils are either unsaturated or saturated. Unsaturated fats can be either monounsaturated or polyunsaturated. Saturated fats, which come mainly from animal sources, increase cholesterol levels. It's best to stay away from these. Tropical oils, such as coconut and palm are non-animal saturated fats - but are so healthy for you, that the benefits outweigh the disadvantages.

Margarine and vegetable shortening are hydrogenated oils, unsaturated fats that have been chemically changed from liquid state into solids by having additional hydrogen atoms pumped into them, thus creating trans-fatty acids. BEWARE! These are the most unhealthful types of fat, and are the number one cause of heart disease. STAY AWAY FROM THESE!

As a *Fun, Fit Foodie*, your goal is to reduce the levels of LDL (bad) cholesterol without lowering the (good) HDL cholesterol. To achieve this, you've got to stick with monounsaturated fats. The most widely used oils that are high in monounsaturated fat are olive oil, canola oil and peanut oil. Polyunsaturated fats, which can include omega-3 and omega-6 essential fatty acids, are considered to be healthy, and include safflower, and grape seed oil. Oils high in omega-3 rich polyunsaturated fat, such as walnut oil, flaxseed oil and canola oil, are a good addition to the diet, since our bodies require omega-3s for good health, but cannot manufacture them. New studies show that incorporating omega-3s into your diet reduces the risk of stroke, heart attack and heart disease, so make sure that you "feed your heart" omega-3s!

> ### *Keep these top oils in your kitchen:*
>
> - Olive oil
> - Safflower oil
> - Grape seed oil
> - Canola oil
> - Peanut oil
> - Pumpkin seed oil
> - Coconut and palm oils

COLD-PRESSED IS BEST!

The way in which the oil you use is extracted also plays a role in how healthy it is. Oil is extracted using one of two methods; mechanical or chemical. Chemical extraction, often called solvent extraction, is the most common and cost-efficient method. It employs high heat and a series of chemical processes, primarily exposure to hexane gas, to remove and refine the oil.

In mechanical extraction, called cold-pressed or expeller-pressed, oil is squeezed from the source, usually with hydraulic presses. This minimal exposure to heat preserves the natural flavor of the oil but limits the yield, making mechanically extracted oils more expensive than chemically extracted oils. We should use only mechanically extracted oils in our diet, in order to maintain the nutrients and health benefits of our oils.

WHICH OILS CAN TAKE THE HEAT?

Each kind of oil is unique, with different nutritional makeup, distinct flavors, and even different smoke points, making some oils more appropriate than others for certain cooking situations.

In cooking, don't overheat oil past its smoke point. If you do, you can cause it to have an odd flavor, and lessen its nutritional value. The worst part of overheating oil is that it can turn the once-healthy oil into a trans-fat-laden heart-disease machine.

Good, all-purpose cooking oils are those that can take high temperatures. Choose from canola, sunflower and peanut oils for high-heat uses, such as searing and frying. Medium-high heat oils are good for baking, sautéing and stir-frying; try grape seed, safflower or sunflower oil. For sauces, lower-heat baking and pressure cooking, medium-high heat oils are best. Good choices are olive oil, corn oil, pumpkinseed oil and walnut oil.

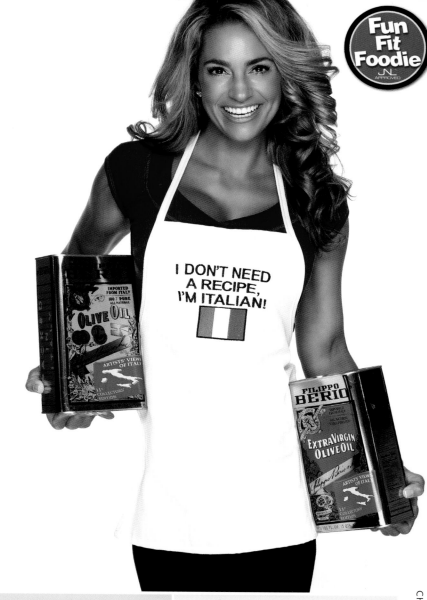

High Temperatures: Searing and Frying	Canola, Sunflower, or Peanut
Medium-High Heat: Baking, Sauteing and Stir Frying	Grapeseed, Safflower, or Sunflower
Lower Heat: Baking and Pressure Cooking	Olive Oil, Pumkinseed, or Walnut Oil

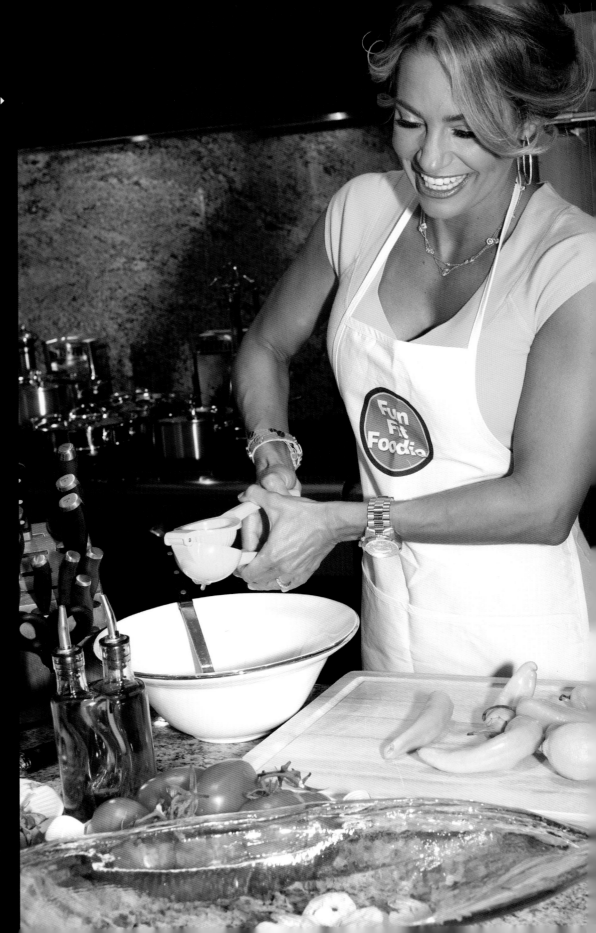

JNL in her home
kitchen, the one
she built, designed,
and now enjoys
cooking in for her
family and friends! ▶

5. THE FFF KITCHEN

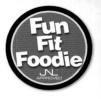

The Fun, Fit Foodie Kitchen: Equipping Your Kitchen With the Right Appliances, Cooking Utensils and Super Food Ingredients!

An artist needs her paint brushes and canvas, an architect needs her scales and drawing boards, and a Fun, Fit Foodie needs her cooking utensils and appliances! Below is my list of must-haves in the kitchen, to equip and awaken your inner chef.

- Copper pots in a range of sizes
- Nonstick skillets (to eliminate the need for excess oil)
- Strainer
- Blender
- Great set of knives
- Wood cutting board-for fruits and veggies
- Plastic cutting board-for meats, as it's more sanitary
- Electric Wine Opener
- Wine Decanter (I like Vinturini)
- Steamer
- Rice Cooker
- Pressure Cooker (I like Wolfgang Puck's)*
- Heat-proof spatulas and wooden spoons
- Measuring cups and spoons

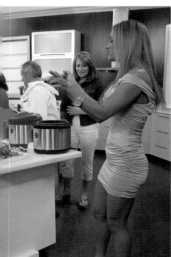
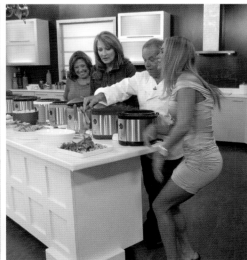
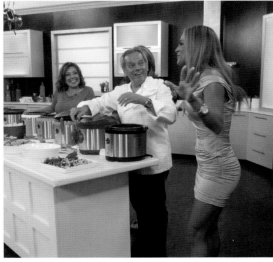

*JNL joins legendary "Celebrity Chef to the Stars" Wolfgang Puck on HSN (Home Shopping Network).

JNL-Approved
Fun, Fit Foodie Grocery List!

Having a well-stocked pantry will prevent the need for fast food and allow you to prepare healthy, Fun, Fit Foodie meals every day.

FRESH OR FROZEN

PROTEINS

- ☐ Lean cuts of beef such as top sirloin, flank steak, eye of round and/or beef tenderloin
- ☐ Extra lean ground beef, turkey or chicken (less than 5 % fat)
- ☐ Turkey breast slices or cutlets (fresh meat, not deli cuts)
- ☐ Boneless, skinless chicken breast
- ☐ Solid light water packed tuna, sodium-reduced if possible (light tuna contains less mercury than albacore tuna)
- ☐ Wild, fresh or frozen fish such as salmon, sea bass or halibut (not farmed)
- ☐ Fresh or frozen shrimp
- ☐ Protein powder
- ☐ Egg whites and/or whole eggs
- ☐ Fibrous Carbs
- ☐ Leaf lettuce (green leaf, red leaf, leaf, romaine)
- ☐ Broccoli
- ☐ Asparagus
- ☐ String beans
- ☐ Spinach
- ☐ Bell peppers
- ☐ Brussels sprouts
- ☐ Cauliflower
- ☐ Celery

OTHER PRODUCE

- ☐ Cucumbers
- ☐ Onions
- ☐ Garlic
- ☐ Tomatoes
- ☐ Zucchini
- ☐ Fruit such as bananas, apples, grapefruit, peaches, strawberries, blueberries, raspberries
- ☐ Lemons or limes
- ☐ Fresh herbs such as basil, coriander, mint and parsley

DAIRY & EGGS

- ☐ Low-fat cottage cheese
- ☐ Eggs
- ☐ Skim milk
- ☐ Reduced fat cheeses such as Swiss, feta and blue cheese (in moderation)

SHELF STABLE

COMPLEX CARBS

- ☐ Whole grain breakfast cereals such as Oatmeal (Old Fashioned or Quick Oats), Multigrain hot cereal, oat bran cereal and/or cream of wheat
- ☐ Sweet Potatoes or yams
- ☐ Potatoes (red, baking, new)
- ☐ Dried beans (pinto, black, kidney)
- ☐ Whole wheat pasta
- ☐ Brown rice (preferably; alternates would include white, Arborio, and wild rice)
- ☐ Barley

HEALTHY FATS

- ☐ Olive oil, canola oil or safflower oil
- ☐ Unrefined coconut oil
- ☐ Natural-style peanut butter
- ☐ Nuts (peanuts, almonds and walnuts)
- ☐ Flaxseed oil

BEVERAGES

- ☐ Bottled water
- ☐ Crystal Light
- ☐ Teas including green tea, white tea and herbal teas
- ☐ Pomegranate juice

CONDIMENTS & MISC.

- ☐ Fat–free mayonnaise
- ☐ Reduced sodium soy sauce
- ☐ Reduced sodium teriyaki sauce
- ☐ Vinegars such as balsamic, white wine, cider and red wine
- ☐ Salsa
- ☐ Dried herbs and spices such as ground cumin, chili powder, ground cinnamon, dried oregano and thyme leaves
- ☐ Mrs. Dash and other salt free seasonings
- ☐ Steak sauce
- ☐ Honey
- ☐ Chili paste
- ☐ Mustard
- ☐ Extracts (vanilla, almond, etc.)
- ☐ Low sodium vegetable, beef or chicken broth
- ☐ Plain or reduced sodium canned tomatoes; sauce, puree, paste
- ☐ Canned light (lite) coconut milk

JNL in Kingston, Jamaica enjoying a fresh a cold organic coconut water right off the truck!

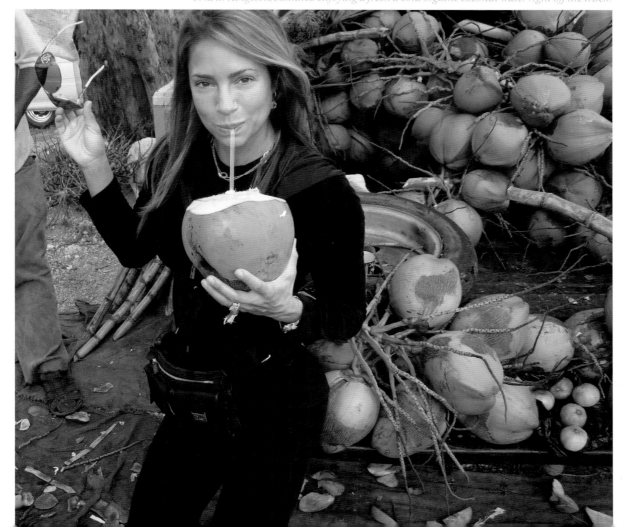

JNL APPROVED LIST OF BRANDS AND FOOD INGREDIENTS

There are just some phenomenal brands of foods that are always going to be staples in my *Fun, Fit Foodie* lifestyle. Here is the "master shopping list" that you can go to in a hurry, and know that you are buying the right stuff for your heart, your mind, and your body!

- ☐ Nutiva Raw Organic Virgin Coconut Oil
- ☐ Artisana Raw Organic Coconut Butter
- ☐ Dove Chocolate
- ☐ BSN Lean Dessert Protein
- ☐ Quaker Oatmeal
- ☐ Campbell's Healthy Choice Soups
- ☐ Natural Oven's Multi-Grain Stay Trim, 100% Whole Grain, Multigrain or Mild Rye
- ☐ Oroweat 100% Whole Wheat, Whole Grain or any Light variety
- ☐ Healthy Choice 100% Whole Grain
- ☐ Brownberry 100% Whole Grain

- ☐ Alvarado Street Bakery Sprouted Bread
- ☐ Trader Joe's Sprouted Breads
- ☐ Arnold Bakery Carb Counting Wheat
- ☐ Sara Lee 100% Whole Wheat or Multi-Grain
- ☐ Baker's Inn 100% Whole Wheat
- ☐ Earth Grain's 100% Whole Wheat
- ☐ Bohemian Hearth 100% Whole Wheat
- ☐ Healthy Life All Varieties
- ☐ La Tortilla Factory Original Low Whole Wheat
- ☐ Trader Joe's Low Carb Flour or Whole Wheat Tortillas
- ☐ Alvarado Street Bakery
- ☐ Ezekiel Sprouted Tortillas
- ☐ Eddie's Whole Wheat Spaghetti
- ☐ Trader Joe's Whole Wheat Pasta
- ☐ Westbrae Natural Whole Wheat or Spinach Spaghetti
- ☐ Hodgson Mill Whole Wheat Spaghetti
- ☐ Prince Healthy Harvest Whole Wheat Blend Pasta
- ☐ Smucker's Simply Fruit or Sugar-Free
- ☐ Sorrell Ridge 100% Fruit

- ☐ Knott's Light
- ☐ Trader Joe's Organic Fruit Spreads
- ☐ Health Valley Fat-Free Cookies (limit to 3), Regular (limit to 1), Biscotti Style (limit to 2) or Café Creations (limit to 1)
- ☐ Hains Kidz Animal Cookies (limit to 10)
- ☐ Pamela's Brand - all varieties (limit to 1)
- ☐ Natural Oven's Chip-Mate or Chocolate Raspberry Cookies (limit to 1)
- ☐ Kashi
- ☐ Nature's Path
- ☐ Health Valley
- ☐ Fiber One or All-Bran
- ☐ Shredded Wheat
- ☐ Wheat Chex
- ☐ Grape Nuts (limit to 1/2 cup portion)
- ☐ Grape Nut Flakes
- ☐ Cheerios
- ☐ Bran Flakes
- ☐ Barbara's Bakery
- ☐ Uncle Sam's Cereal
- ☐ Quaker Oat Bran or Crunchy C

ADDITIONAL JNL FUN FIT FOOD APPROVED WEBSITES:

- American Heart Association Go Red for Women **Goredforwomen**.org
- **Kraft**.com
- **Nabisco**.com
- **Carnationbreakfastessentials**.com
- **Sargento**.com
- **Boboli**.com
- **Stouffers**.com
- **Wholefoods**.com

Following My Fun, Fit Foodie Recipes

These recipes represent some of my favorite foods to eat. Here are some helpful tips to ensure that you have success at home with my Fun, Fit Foodie recipes:

- Wherever you see the volume "JAT," it means "Just a Touch" and is the same as a "pinch." In some cases I use JAT to control the amount of sugar and sodium added to a recipe. For salt free seasonings, please adjust the amounts to suit your own personal taste.
- When I call for eggs, I assume you are using large-size eggs.
- Frozen, unsweetened IQF (individually quick frozen) berries are a great option when fresh berries are out of season, arrange on a baking sheet lined with paper towel to thaw and use wherever fresh berries are called for in a recipe.
- When I call for extra lean ground beef, I prefer that you choose grass fed, antibiotic free beef that is less than 5% fat.

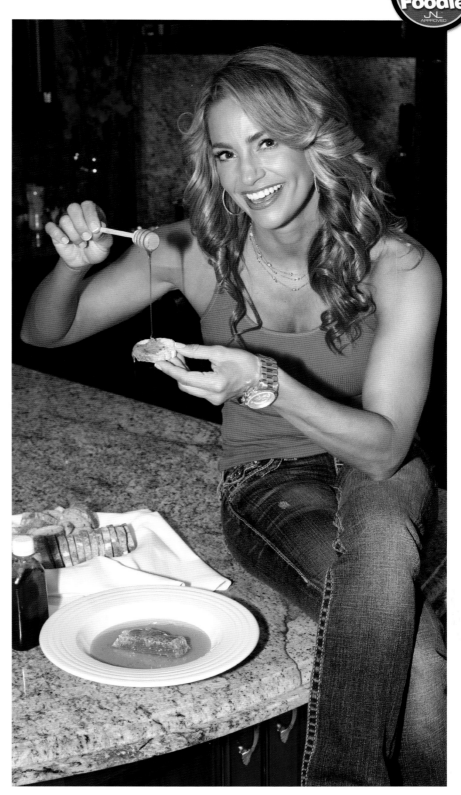

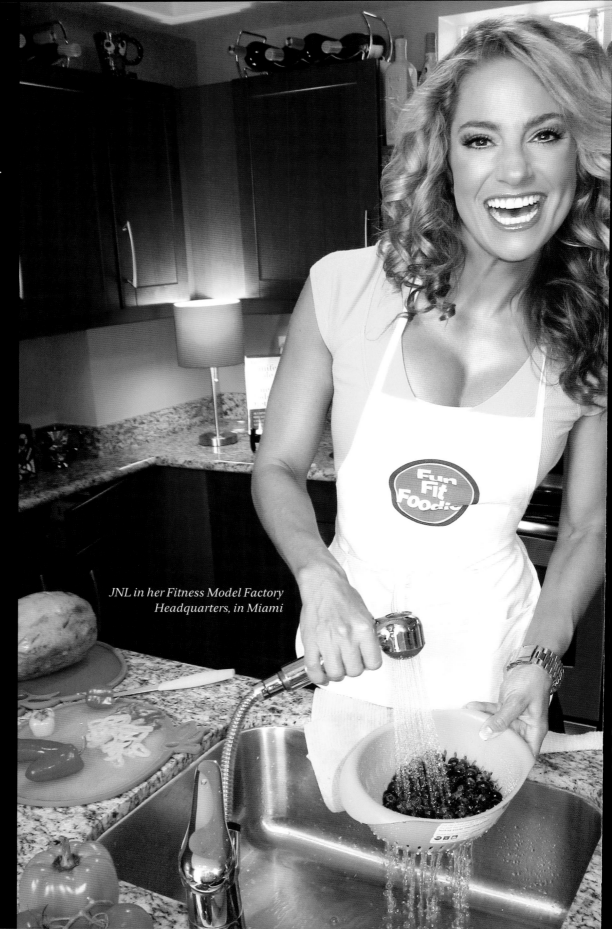

Breakfast is the most important meal of the day. Start your day right with a metabolism boosting, fat burning and calorie-torching breakfast.

6. BREAKFAST

JNL in her Fitness Model Factory Headquarters, in Miami

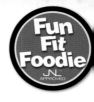

Southwest Veggie Scramble

Serve this easy scramble with complex carbs such as a slice of whole grain toast and ½ cup serving of high fiber cereal. Add some fresh fruit to your cereal to boost your morning intake of antioxidants.

INGREDIENTS:

- ½ tsp canola oil
- ¾ cup mixed veggies (such as fresh spinach, mushrooms and green pepper)
- 6 cherry tomatoes, halved
- 3 egg whites
- 1 whole egg
- 1 tbsp skim milk
- JAT black pepper and cayenne pepper

DIRECTIONS:

1. Coat a skillet lightly with the canola oil. Add the vegetables and sauté for 2 to 3 minutes or until tender. Add the cherry tomatoes, sauté for 2 minutes.

2. While the vegetables are sautéing, beat the eggs with milk in a small bowl. Add black and cayenne pepper to taste.

3. Pour the eggs into the pan and cook, stirring, until eggs are scrambled and cooked to your preference. Serves 1.

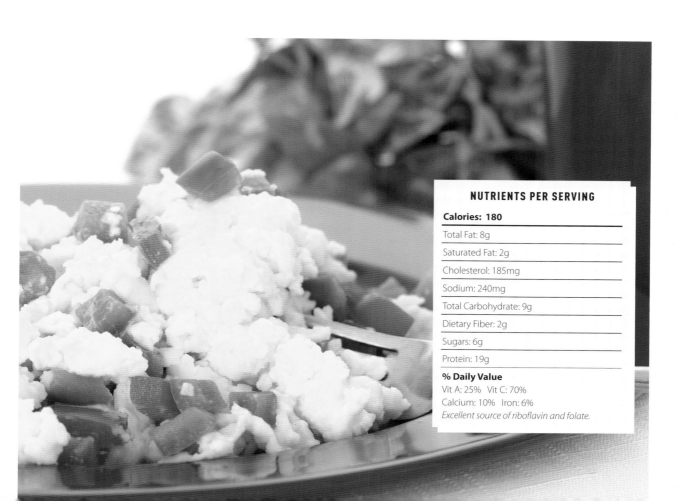

NUTRIENTS PER SERVING

Calories: 180

Total Fat: 8g	
Saturated Fat: 2g	
Cholesterol: 185mg	
Sodium: 240mg	
Total Carbohydrate: 9g	
Dietary Fiber: 2g	
Sugars: 6g	
Protein: 19g	

% Daily Value
Vit A: 25%   Vit C: 70%
Calcium: 10% Iron: 6%
Excellent source of riboflavin and folate.

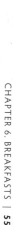

"Knock Your Wig Off" Waffles

Tender apple and cinnamon flavored waffles that can be topped with fresh fruit and nonfat yogurt for a wholesome breakfast. The soy flour can be replaced with rice or potato flour if you are intolerant or allergic to soy.

INGREDIENTS:

- 2 egg whites
- JAT salt
- JAT cream of tartar
- ½ cup non-fat Greek-style yogurt
- ¼ cup unsweetened applesauce
- 2 tbsp skim milk
- 1 tsp raw honey
- 1 tsp vanilla extract
- ¼ cup plus 2 tbsp whole-wheat pastry flour
- ¼ cup graham flour
- ¼ cup soy flour
- 2 tbsp wheat bran
- 1 ½ tsp baking powder
- ½ tsp ground cinnamon

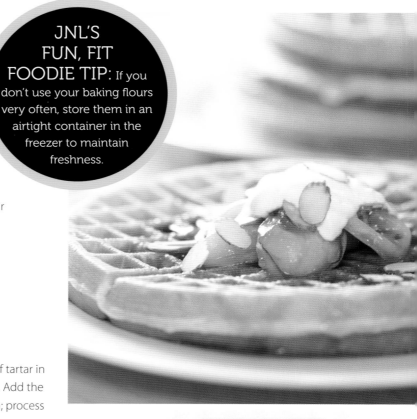

JNL'S FUN, FIT FOODIE TIP: If you don't use your baking flours very often, store them in an airtight container in the freezer to maintain freshness.

DIRECTIONS:

1. Combine the egg whites, salt, and cream of tartar in a blender; blend for 1 minute or until fluffy. Add the yogurt, applesauce, milk, honey and vanilla; process until smooth.

2. In a separate bowl sift the whole-wheat, graham and soy flours with the bran, baking powder and cinnamon. Add the dry ingredients to the blender and process until well combined.

3. Bake in a waffle iron according to the manufacturer's directions. Makes five square Belgian-style waffles. (Recipe doubles easily.)

NUTRIENTS PER SERVING
(1 waffle)

Calories: 110	
Total Fat: 0g	
Saturated Fat: 0g	
Cholesterol: 0mg	
Sodium: 360mg	
Total Carbohydrate: 19g	
Dietary Fiber: 4g	
Sugars: 5g	
Protein: 8g	

% Daily Value
Vit A: 0%   Vit C: 0%
Calcium: 6%   Iron: 6%
Excellent source of riboflavin and folate.

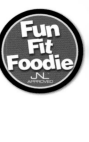

Egg Bruschetta

INGREDIENTS:

- 2 or 3 ripe tomatoes, thickly sliced
- 2 large cloves garlic
- 4 slices whole-grain toast
- 4 eggs
- 2 tsp olive oil
- JAT sea salt and freshly ground pepper

DIRECTIONS:

1. Broil the tomato slices; keep warm. Lightly rub the garlic onto the toast (for more garlic flavor, rub longer).

2. Meanwhile, fry the eggs in the olive oil until cooked to your preferred doneness. To assemble, layer tomatoes onto each slice of garlic toast. Season with salt and pepper to taste. Top with the fried eggs and serve immediately. Serves 4.

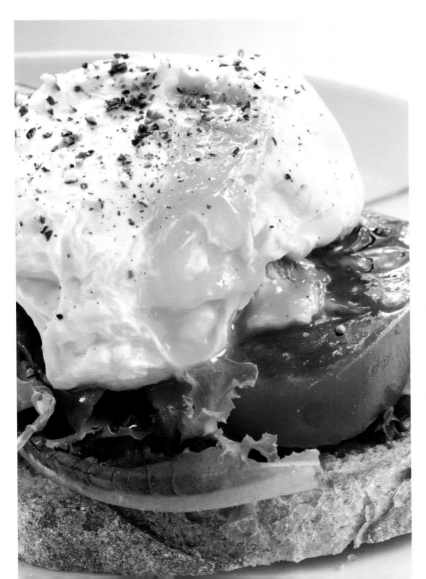

NUTRIENTS PER SERVING
(1 toast with egg)

Calories: 190

Total Fat: 8g	
Saturated Fat: 2g	
Cholesterol: 185mg	
Sodium: 310mg	
Total Carbohydrate: 22g	
Dietary Fiber: 4g	
Sugars: 6g	
Protein: 11g	

% Daily Value
Vit A: 0%   Vit C: 20%
Calcium: 20%   Iron: 20%

Protein-Packed Blueberry Pancakes

Everybody loves a stack of pancakes in the morning. These pancakes get a boost of protein from the cottage cheese and egg whites. Serve warm, topped with maple syrup, fruit, or my personal favorite – almond butter!

INGREDIENTS:

- 1 cup rolled oats
- 1 cup fat-free cottage cheese
- 6 egg whites (about ¾ cup)
- 2 tsp agave nectar or honey
- ½ tsp vanilla extract
- ½ tsp ground cinnamon
- ½ cup fresh or thawed, frozen blueberries

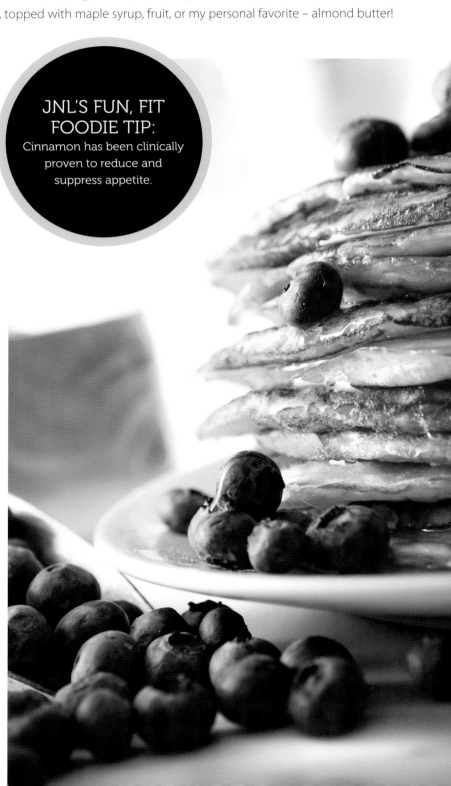

JNL'S FUN, FIT FOODIE TIP:
Cinnamon has been clinically proven to reduce and suppress appetite.

DIRECTIONS:

1. Combine oats, cottage cheese, egg whites, agave nectar, vanilla and cinnamon in a blender; blend for 30 seconds or until well-combined and smooth. Gently stir in the blueberries.

2. Preheat a non-stick skillet or griddle over medium heat; coat lightly with cooking spray. Scoop 1/4 cup portions of the batter onto the hot pan without crowding the pan.

3. Cook for about 3 minutes or until the edges start to bubble. Flip the pancakes; cook for 2 minutes, or until golden brown. Repeat with remaining batter, using additional cooking spray as needed. Serves 4 (makes about 12 pancakes).

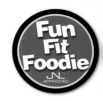

Greek Omelet with Feta Cheese

A little feta cheese goes a long way in this tasty omelet. Serve with toasted whole-wheat bread, and you'll have a perfectly balanced Fun, Fit Foodie breakfast!

INGREDIENTS:

- 5 egg whites
- 1 whole egg
- ½ tsp Mrs. Dash Tomato Basil and Garlic Salt-Free seasoning
- ½ cup mixed chopped tomatoes, green peppers and onion
- 2 tbsp crumbled reduced-fat feta cheese

DIRECTIONS:

1. Coat a large skillet with cooking spray and set over medium heat.
2. Whisk the eggs with the seasoning. Pour into the skillet; cook for about 4 minutes until omelet is just cooked completely through. Sprinkle the vegetables and cheese over one side of the omelet; fold the other side over to enclose the filling. Serves 2.

◀ **NUTRIENTS PER SERVING**
(3 pancakes)

Calories: 160

Total Fat: 1.5g	
Saturated Fat: 0g	
Cholesterol: 5mg	
Sodium: 290mg	
Total Carbohydrate: 23g	
Dietary Fiber: 3g	
Sugars: 8g	
Protein: 14g	

% Daily Value
Vit A: 2%   Vit C: 4%
Calcium: 4%   Iron: 6%

NUTRIENTS PER SERVING
(½ omelet)

Calories: 110

Total Fat: 4.5g	
Saturated Fat: 2g	
Cholesterol: 100mg	
Sodium: 270mg	
Total Carbohydrate: 3g	
Dietary Fiber: 0g	
Sugars: 2g	
Protein: 14g	

% Daily Value
Vit A: 0%   Vit C: 25%
Calcium: 6%   Iron: 2%
Excellent source of riboflavin.

Goof-Proof Grab & Go Breakfast Burrito

If you think whipping up a breakfast burrito in the morning will take too much time, think again! I've simplified the steps so you can make it, and then make it out the door on time. Pre-chop your vegetables and have the egg mixture ready to go in the fridge. Any leftover burritos, I wrap in aluminum foil to re-heat and eat later as a snack.

INGREDIENTS:

- 2 tsp olive oil, divided
- 2 tbsp finely diced white onion
- ½ cup sliced mushrooms
- 1 to 2 jalapeño peppers (or more depending on how spicy you want your burrito to be)
- 1 cup baby spinach leaves
- 2 tbsp chopped tomatoes
- 6 whole eggs
- 6 egg whites
- ¼ cup crumbled reduced-fat feta cheese
- 1 tbsp chopped fresh cilantro (optional)
- 6 medium (8-inch) whole-wheat tortillas

DIRECTIONS:

1. Lightly coat medium-size skillet with half of the olive oil. Place over medium high heat. Add onion and cook, for 2 minutes or until almost transparent. Add mushrooms and jalapenos and cook for 1 minute or until tender. Add baby spinach leaves and tomatoes, cooking for 1 minute or until spinach is wilted. Scrape into a bowl.

2. Whisk whole eggs with egg whites until combined. Reduce the heat under the skillet to medium. Pour in the eggs. Cook for 1 minute without stirring; add vegetable mixture. Cook, stirring, until eggs are cooked through and fluffy. Sprinkle with crumbled feta cheese. Sprinkle with cilantro (if using). Spoon the egg mixture onto tortillas, roll up to enclose filling. Serves 6 (makes 6 burritos).

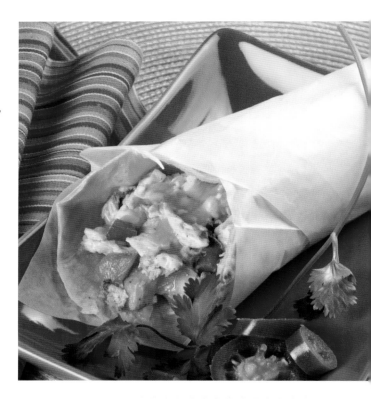

NUTRIENTS PER SERVING
(1 burrito)

Calories: 220

Total Fat: 10g	
Saturated Fat: 2.5g	
Cholesterol: 190mg	
Sodium: 400mg	
Total Carbohydrate: 16g	
Dietary Fiber: 3g	
Sugars: 1g	
Protein: 14g	

% Daily Value
Vit A: 10%   Vit C: 10%
Calcium: 6%   Iron: 6%
Excellent source of folate.

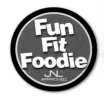

Chai Cream of Wheat Topped with Walnuts

This is an excellent hot breakfast cereal and a nice change from oatmeal. I love the fact that you get nearly half the daily recommended allowance of iron from one serving of Cream of Wheat. Top with walnuts, you are also getting heart-healthy fats and muscle- building protein. Dig in!

INGREDIENTS:

- 3 tbsp Cream of Wheat Cereal (non-instant)
- ¾ cup water
- JAT ground cinnamon
- JAT ground coriander
- JAT ground cardamom
- JAT turmeric
- 1 tbsp chopped toasted walnuts
- 2 tsp honey

DIRECTIONS:

1. Prepare the cereal as directed on the package instructions. Stir in the cinnamon, coriander, cardamom and turmeric, adjusting seasonings to taste.

2. Spoon into a bowl and sprinkle with walnuts. Drizzle honey on top. Serves 1.

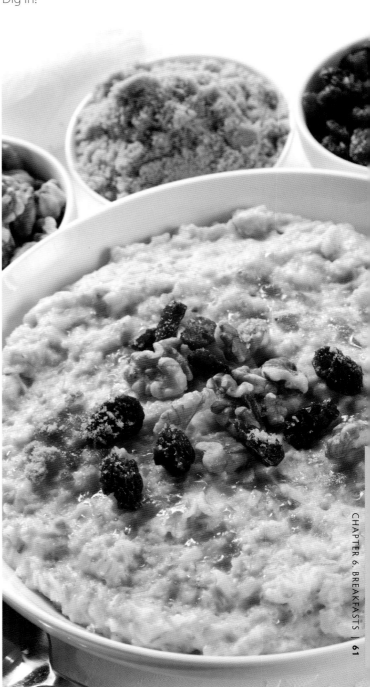

NUTRIENTS PER SERVING

Calories: 220

Total Fat: 4.5g
Saturated Fat: .5g
Cholesterol: 0mg
Sodium: 0mg
Total Carbohydrate: 38g
Dietary Fiber: 2g
Sugars: 12g
Protein: 5g

% Daily Value
Vit A: 0%   Vit C: 0%
Calcium: 2%   Iron: 25%

JNL's Fun, Fit Foodie Ranchero Breakfast Bowl

Instead of high-starch white potatoes, I use brown rice in this recipe. When I've got a long morning commute, I put this in a Tupperware bowl and enjoy my breakfast "to go." This hearty combo will get your body and your taste buds into 5th gear! Vrrrommmm!!!

INGREDIENTS:

- 5 egg whites
- 1 whole egg
- ¼ cup drained and rinsed canned black beans
- ¼ cup drained and rinsed canned pinto beans
- ¼ cup diced mixed bell peppers (red, orange, green and/or yellow)
- 2 tbsp salsa
- 1 cup hot cooked brown rice.
- Fat free sour cream (optional)
- Chopped chives (optional)

JNL'S FUN, FIT FOODIE TIP: Invest in a rice cooker, so you can always have hot, fresh brown rice ready when you need it, without the fuss.

DIRECTIONS:

1. Whisk eggs whites with the whole egg until combined. Coat a medium-sized skillet with cooking spray and set over medium-high heat. Add eggs and cook, stirring, until just beginning to set. Add beans, and bell peppers to eggs; cook, stirring, until cooked to preferred doneness.

2. Place the rice in a bowl or container. Spoon the scrambled egg mixture over top. Spoon the salsa over the egg mixture. Garnish with sour cream and chives (if using). Serves 2.

NUTRIENTS PER SERVING

Calories: 240	
Total Fat: 3.5g	
Saturated Fat: 1g	
Cholesterol: 95mg	
Sodium: 450mg	
Total Carbohydrate: 34g	
Dietary Fiber: 4g	
Sugars: 3g	
Protein: 17g	

% Daily Value
Vit A: 2%   Vit C: 40%
Calcium: 6%   Iron: 8%
Excellent source of riboflavin, folate and selenium.

Protein-Packed Sweet Potato Hash

This breakfast is so rich, sweet and filling, it feels like a feast fit for a queen! The sweet potato is packed full of vitamin C, fiber and beta-carotene, all excellent for your overall health. It serves up like a casserole, thick and delicious.

INGREDIENTS:

- 1 medium sweet potato, cut into equal, bite-sized pieces
- ¼ cup water
- 1 scoop vanilla protein powder
- 2 tbsp chopped pecans
- JAT ground cinnamon
- JAT ground nutmeg
- 1 tsp honey

DIRECTIONS:

1. Combine the sweet potato and water in a microwave-safe bowl. Microwave on High for about 4 minutes or until potatoes cooked through. Stir in the protein powder, pecans, cinnamon and nutmeg. Transfer to a serving bowl. Drizzle with the honey. Serves 1.

NUTRIENTS PER SERVING

Calories: 400

Total Fat: 14g	
Saturated Fat: 2g	
Cholesterol: 50mg	
Sodium: 160mg	
Total Carbohydrate: 42g	
Dietary Fiber: 6g	
Sugars: 17g	
Protein: 24g	

% Daily Value
Vit A: 120%   Vit C: 35%
Calcium: 20%   Iron: 10%
Excellent source of thiamin and riboflavin.

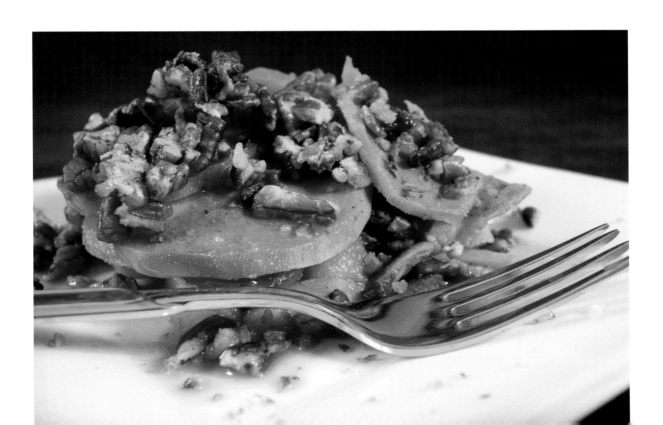

60 Second Fun, Fit and FAST Foodie Breakfast

I know we all have those super rammed-jammed, hectic mornings, but we must eat our breakfast. Reserve this breakfast for when your morning is REALLY busy! Plan ahead and prepare the hardboiled eggs the night before. Voila! A complete breakfast, ready in under a minute that will fuel you for most of your morning.

INGREDIENTS:

- 3 hard boiled eggs
- ½ cup skim milk
- ½ cup high fiber bran cereal (such as All Bran Fiber Buds)
- ¼ cup fresh or thawed, frozen blueberries

DIRECTIONS:

1. Peel the eggs. Remove the yolks from two of the hardboiled eggs and reserve for another purpose. (You'll be eating the whites of all three, but only one yolk.) Pour milk over cereal, top with berries. Serves 1.

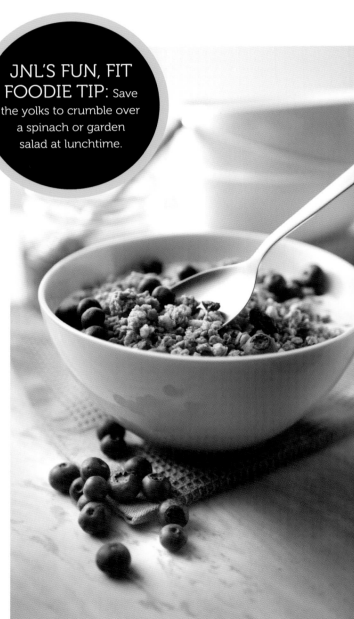

JNL'S FUN, FIT FOODIE TIP: Save the yolks to crumble over a spinach or garden salad at lunchtime.

NUTRIENTS PER SERVING

Calories: 280	
Total Fat: 7g	
Saturated Fat: 2g	
Cholesterol: 205mg	
Sodium: 530mg	
Total Carbohydrate: 48g	
Dietary Fiber: 20g	
Sugars: 23g	
Protein: 21g	

% Daily Value
Vit A: 25%   Vit C: 25%
Calcium: 30%   Iron: 40%
Excellent source of riboflavin, niacin, vitamin B6, folate, vitamin B12, vitamin D, magnesium, selenium, and zinc.

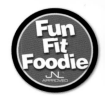

Fitness Model Enchiladas

Because it was such a hit, I borrowed this recipe from my Fitness Model book. It's a fun and fit recipe that any foodie would love! The avocado is great for your heart health, and also for your hair, skin, and nails. And the whole-wheat tortillas give you the morning carbs and fiber your body needs to kick-start the day off right.

INGREDIENTS:

- 3 egg whites
- 1 whole egg,
- 1 ½ tbsp reduced-fat shredded cheddar cheese
- 2 small whole-wheat tortillas
- ¼ cup sliced avocado
- ¼ cup salsa

DIRECTIONS:

1. Lightly coat a small nonstick skillet with cooking spray; place over medium heat. Whisk egg whites with the whole egg until blended. Add to the pan and cook, stirring, until scrambled and cooked to preferred doneness. Sprinkle with shredded cheese.

2. Lightly dampen 2 paper towels and place tortillas between them. Cook tortillas in the microwave for 30 seconds on High or until gently warmed. Divide the scrambled eggs between the tortillas. Top each with an equal portion of the salsa and avocado; roll up to enclose the filling. Serves 1 to 2.

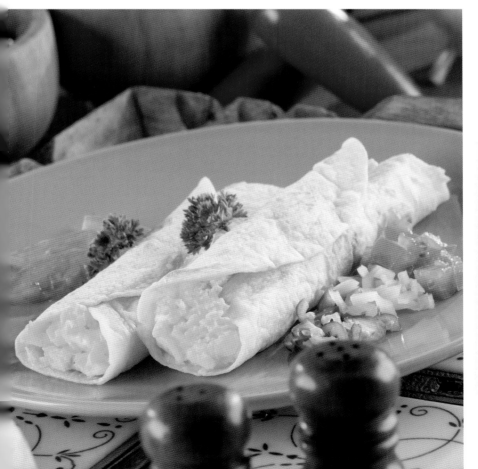

NUTRIENTS PER SERVING
(1 enchilada)

Calories: 200	
Total Fat: 9g	
Saturated Fat: 2g	
Cholesterol: 95mg	
Sodium: 470mg	
Total Carbohydrate: 17g	
Dietary Fiber: 3g	
Sugars: 2g	
Protein: 13g	

% Daily Value
Vit A: 2%   Vit C: 4%
Calcium: 6%   Iron: 2%
Excellent source of folate and selenium.

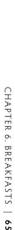

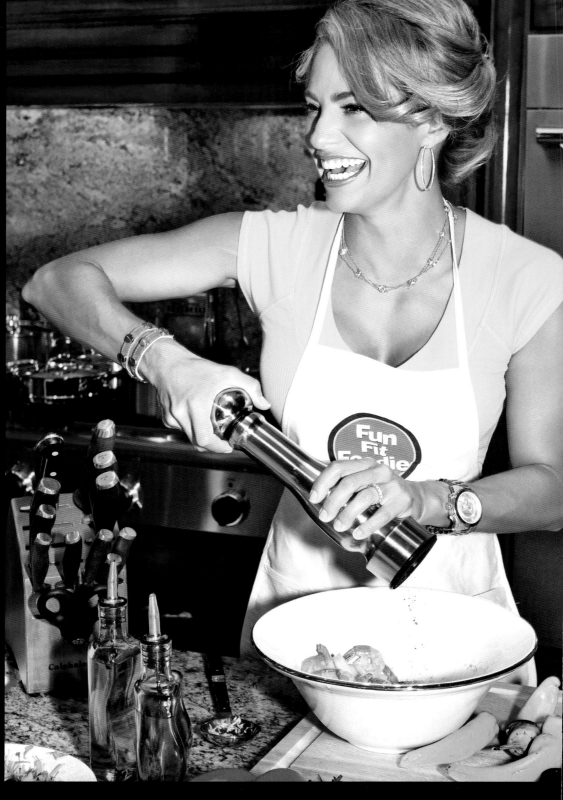

THE FUN, FIT FOODIE LUNCH FORMULA:

Lunch should be the second-biggest meal of your day, after breakfast. Lunch needs to be balanced, to give your healthy and humming body what it needs. You should always include a lean source of protein, a source of fibrous carbs, and also a whole-grain carb, with a touch of a good-for-you fat.

7. LUNCH

"You are NEVER too busy to eat lunch! If you skip it, come late afternoon, your body will crash, setting you up for failure. Pre-pack your Fun, Fit Foodie meal and eat it on the go if you must, or at your desk. If it's a gorgeous day, take a quick break and eat outside, savoring every healthy bite." —JNL

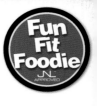

Glorious Grapefruit Chicken Salad

A zesty and refreshing way to fuel you up for the afternoon.

INGREDIENTS:

- 2 cups diced cooked chicken breast
- 1 ½ cups grapefruit segments, chopped
- ¼ cup chopped celery
- 1 scallion, minced
- ¼ cup plain, non-fat yogurt
- ¼ cup fat-free mayonnaise
- ¼ cup fresh parsley, finely chopped
- JAT celery seeds
- 4 cups mixed salad greens
- 8 whole-wheat Melba toasts

JNL'S FUN, FIT FOODIE TIP: Have lean chicken breast always at the ready by poaching or grilling boneless, skinless chicken breasts in batches. Chop and pack into freezer bags; simply grab a bag to thaw in the refrigerator the night before you want to use them.

DIRECTIONS:

1. Toss chicken with the grapefruit, celery and scallion in a large bowl.

2. Blend the yogurt with the mayonnaise, parsley and celery seeds until combined. Add the dressing to the chicken mixture and toss to combine. Spoon the chicken mixture over mixed greens. Serve with melba toast on the side. Serves 4.

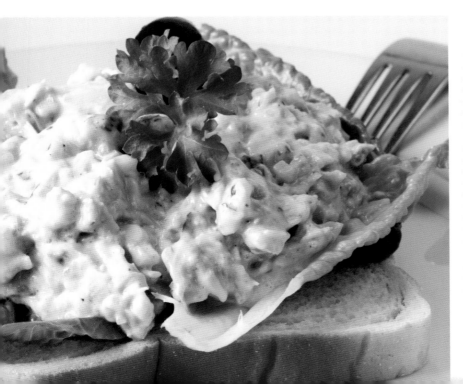

NUTRIENTS PER SERVING
(¼ recipe)

Calories: 210

Total Fat: 2.5g	
Saturated Fat: 1g	
Cholesterol: 60mg	
Sodium: 280mg	
Total Carbohydrate: 22g	
Dietary Fiber: 2g	
Sugars: 3g	
Protein: 26g	

% Daily Value
Vit A: 15%   Vit C: 70%
Calcium: 8%   Iron: 8%
Excellent source of niacin, vitamin B6 and selenium.

Tangy Tuna Melt

This satisfying, fork and knife sandwich contains tuna, which is a source of Omega-3, an essential fatty acid that your healthy body needs. Serve with a side of crunchy vegetable crudités!

INGREDIENTS:

- 2 can (6 oz each) water-packed, sodium-reduced light tuna, drained
- ¼ cup fat-free mayonnaise
- 2 tsp dijon mustard
- JAT freshly ground black pepper
- 1 cup baby spinach
- 4 slices whole grain bread
- 4 slices reduced-fat Swiss cheese

DIRECTIONS:

1. Preheat the broiler or toaster oven. Blend tuna with mayonnaise, mustard and pepper.

2. Lightly toast the bread slices in a toaster. Top each slice of bread with an equal portion of the spinach leaves, tuna salad and sliced cheese.

3. Broil sandwiches for about 1 minute or until cheese melts. Serves 4.

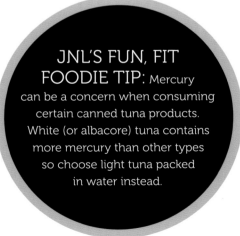

JNL'S FUN, FIT FOODIE TIP: Mercury can be a concern when consuming certain canned tuna products. White (or albacore) tuna contains more mercury than other types so choose light tuna packed in water instead.

NUTRIENTS PER SERVING (1 sandwich)
Calories: 190
Total Fat: 3g
Saturated Fat: 1g
Cholesterol: 35mg
Sodium: 480mg
Total Carbohydrate: 17g
Dietary Fiber: 2g
Sugars: 2g
Protein: 24g

% Daily Value
Vit A: 20%   Vit C: 6%
Calcium: 25%   Iron: 10%

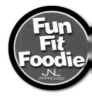

Grilled Citrus Marinated Chicken Breasts with Avocado

Bored with chicken? No longer once you taste my recipe! Serve with a side of steamed brown rice, vegetables or a leafy green salad for a complete meal.

INGREDIENTS:

- 4 boneless, skinless chicken breasts
- 2 pink grapefruits, divided
- 1 navel orange
- 1 lemon
- JAT lemon pepper seasoning
- 1 avocado, sliced

DIRECTIONS:

1. Juice one grapefruit, the orange and lemon; mix well. Pour the fruit juices over the chicken and marinate overnight.

2. Preheat the grill to medium. Sprinkle lemon pepper on marinated breasts. Grill the chicken, turning as needed, for 15 to 20 minutes or until cooked through.

3. Meanwhile, slice the remaining grapefruit; place on the grill and cook, turning once until well marked on each side. Serve chicken on the grilled grapefruit and top with sliced avocado. Serves 4.

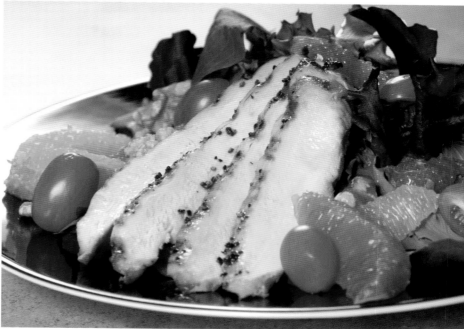

NUTRIENTS PER SERVING
(1 chicken breast with avocado)

Calories: 320

Total Fat: 10g	
Saturated Fat: 2g	
Cholesterol: 105mg	
Sodium: 160mg	
Total Carbohydrate: 12g	
Dietary Fiber: 4g	
Sugars: 5g	
Protein: 44g	

% Daily Value
Vit A: 0%   Vit C: 50%
Calcium: 4%   Iron: 10%
Excellent source of niacin and vitamin B6.

Siciliano (Turkey) Meatballs

One of my favorite memories as a child was sitting around a table enjoying a bowl of spaghetti and meatballs. I've exchanged the high-fat ground beef for low-fat turkey, slashing the calories while keeping the protein high and the taste delicious! Make batches of these meatballs and freeze for spaghetti and meatballs anytime.

INGREDIENTS:

- 4 slices dry or day old whole wheat bread
- ½ cup water
- 4 egg whites
- ¾ cup grated light parmesan cheese
- 2 tsp dried parsley
- 2 tsp dried oregano
- 1 lb lean ground turkey
- 2 cups no added salt, canned diced tomatoes
- 6 cups hot, cooked whole-wheat (or whole-wheat with flax) spaghetti

JNL'S FUN, FIT FOODIE TIP: Yes, you can have carbs, as long as they're the right ones. Use high fiber, whole-wheat or even better, whole-wheat pasta that also contains flax to provide beneficial omega 3 fatty acids. And watch your portion control. A meal-sized serving should be no more than 1 cup of pasta with 4 meatballs and sauce.

DIRECTIONS:

1. Preheat the oven to 350°F. Place the bread into a bowl and pour the water over it. Let stand until the most of the water is absorbed; discard excess water. Break up the bread using your fingertips. Stir in the egg whites, cheese, parsley and oregano. Crumble in the turkey; mix to combine.

2. Lightly coat a cookie sheet with nonstick spray. Roll the mixture into 16 balls and place on the prepared sheet. Bake for 20 to 30 minutes or until meatballs are cooked through. Meanwhile, heat the tomatoes in a saucepan set over medium heat until simmering. Add the meatballs and toss to coat. Serve meatballs and tomatoes over the hot cooked pasta. Serves 6.

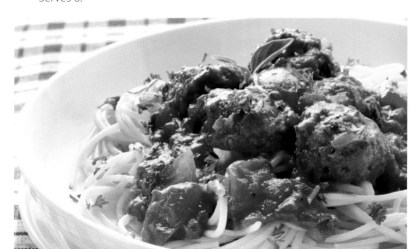

NUTRIENTS PER SERVING
(4 meatballs with sauce and pasta)

Calories: 470

Total Fat: 13g	
Saturated Fat: 2.5g	
Cholesterol: 80mg	
Sodium: 420mg	
Total Carbohydrate: 57mg	
Dietary Fiber: 7g	
Sugars: 4g	
Protein: 33g	

% Daily Value
Vit A: 0%   Vit C: 6%
Calcium: 15%   Iron: 20%
Excellent source of niacin and manganese.

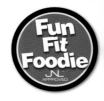

Fun, Fit Foodie Tropical Chicken Salad Sandwich

WOW! Talk about waking up your taste buds with a flavor TKO! Chunks of golden pineapple tossed with succulent, cooked chicken and crisp celery make this recipe the perfect reason to never skip lunch again.

INGREDIENTS:

- 1 cup chopped, cooked boneless, skinless chicken breast
- 1 stalk celery, diced
- 2 tbsp chopped fresh or drained, canned pineapple
- 2 tbsp fat-free mayonnaise
- JAT ground cinnamon
- 4 slices whole-wheat bread

DIRECTIONS:

1. Toss the chicken with the celery, pineapple, mayonnaise and cinnamon. Divide the chicken mixture between two slices of bread. Cap with remaining bread slices.

2. Lightly coat a skillet with nonstick cooking spray; set over medium heat. Add the sandwiches and cook for 2 to 3 minutes per side or until lightly browned. Serves 2.

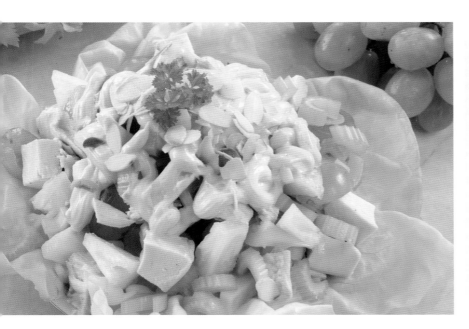

NUTRIENTS PER SERVING
(1 sandwich)

Calories: 390	
Total Fat: 10g	
Saturated Fat: 1g	
Cholesterol: 65mg	
Sodium: 660mg	
Total Carbohydrate: 44g	
Dietary Fiber: 6g	
Sugars: 8g	
Protein: 31g	

% Daily Value
Vit A: 0% Vit C: 4%
Calcium: 6% Iron: 15%
Excellent source of niacin, vitamin B6 and selenium

Whole-Wheat Wrap with Blackened Shrimp

I love Cajun cooking, because it's as colorful and spicy as the city of New Orleans. I whip up this up in honor of Mardi Gras. Instead of making it as a typical Po'boy, I replaced the doughy submarine hoagie buns with a lighter whole-wheat wrap. Serve with a green salad on the side, and you are set for a healthy celebration in your mouth and tummy!

INGREDIENTS

- 1 lb large raw shrimp, peeled and de-veined
- 1 tbsp Mrs. Dash(R) Extra Spicy salt-free seasoning
- 2 tbsp lime juice, divided
- ¼ cup fat-free mayonnaise
- 2 tbsp dijon mustard
- 4 large whole-wheat tortillas or wraps
- 1 each red, yellow and green peppers, seeded and sliced
- 1 tsp garlic paste

JNL'S FUN, FIT FOODIE TIP:
Shrimp provides low-fat and low-calorie protein. Shrimp also contains selenium, a micronutrient that neutralizes the injurious effects of free radicals, which are among the main causes of cancer and other degenerative diseases.

DIRECTIONS:

1. Toss shrimp with seasoning in a small bowl. Drizzle with half of the lime juice. Cover and marinate in the fridge for 1 hour. Blend the mayonnaise with the mustard and remaining lime juice. Set aside.

2. Lightly coat a skillet with nonstick cooking spray and place over medium-high heat. Add shrimp; stir-fry for 2 to 3 minutes or until shrimp are pink. Remove the shrimp to a bowl, cover to keep warm. Reduce the heat to medium; add peppers and stir-fry for about 5 minutes. Add the garlic paste and stir-fry for another 5 minutes or until peppers are cooked, but still a tad crunchy.

3. Spread the mayonnaise mixture over the wraps. Divide the peppers and shrimp between the tortillas. Roll up to enclose the filling. Serves 4.

NUTRIENTS PER SERVING
(1 wrap)

Calories: 280

Total Fat: 5g	
Saturated Fat: 1g	
Cholesterol: 55mg	
Sodium: 630mg	
Total Carbohydrate: 36mg	
Dietary Fiber: 5g	
Sugars: 3g	
Protein: 12g	

% Daily Value
Vit A: 0%   Vit C: 260%
Calcium: 20%   Iron: 15%

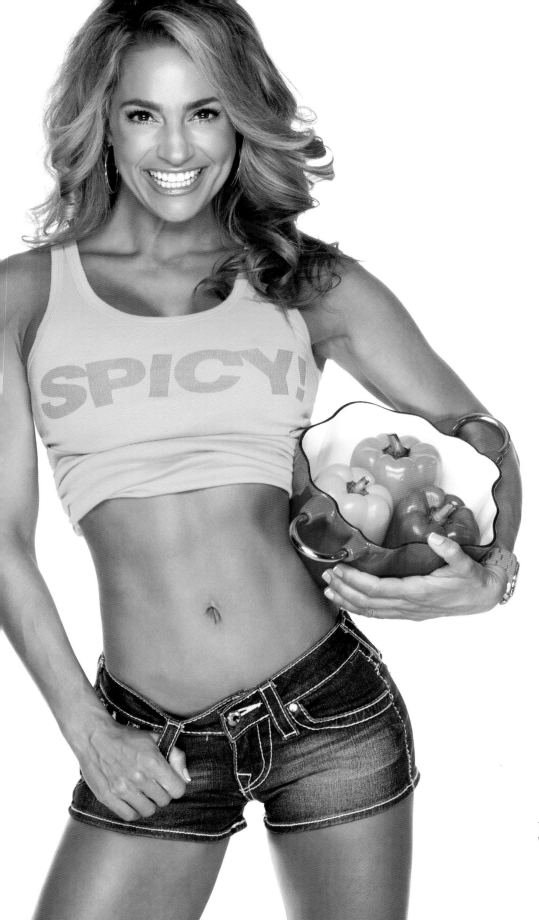

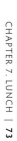

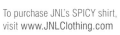

To purchase JNL's SPICY shirt,
visit www.JNLClothing.com

"Latina Loca" Beef Bowl Salad

Living in Miami, the spices and creative food influences never stop! "Latina Loca " is the perfect mix of sizzling lean red meat for protein and iron, served on top of high fiber brown rice, and then topped with cool, heart-friendly condiments such as guacamole and crisp salad, all served up neatly in one bowl! A great way to use up leftovers; food can't get any better or easier than this!

INGREDIENTS:

- 1 cup cooked lean antibiotic-free, grass fed ground beef, about 4% fat
- JAT Mrs. Dash Southwest Chipotle seasoning
- 1 cup hot, cooked brown rice
- 2 cups shredded lettuce
- 2 tbsp salsa
- 2 tbsp HOLY MOLY Guacamole *(see recipe on page 121)*
- 2 tbsp diced tomatoes
- 2 tbsp fat-free sour cream

DIRECTIONS:

1. Warm beef with seasoning in a skillet or in the microwave. Layer the ingredients into two bowls in the following order: rice, beef, lettuce, salsa, guacamole, tomatoes and sour cream. Serves 2.

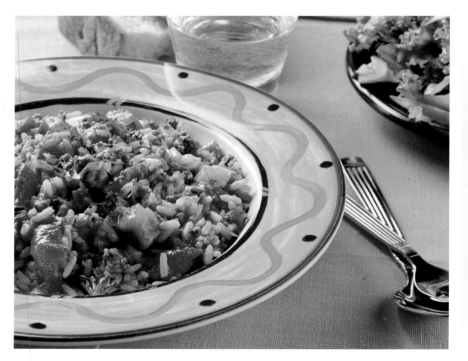

NUTRIENTS PER SERVING

Calories: 590	
Total Fat: 21g	
Saturated Fat: 8g	
Cholesterol: 100mg	
Sodium: 370mg	
Total Carbohydrate: 53g	
Dietary Fiber: 5g	
Sugars: 5g	
Protein: 44g	

% Daily Value
Vit A: 15%   Vit C: 20%
Calcium: 20%   Iron: 25%
Excellent source of riboflavin, thiamin, niacin, vitamin B6, selenium and zinc.

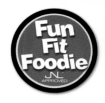

Siciliano Grilled Chicken Deli Flatbread Sandwich

An Italian girl loves her meat, bread and cheese! This is a healthy rendition of one of my favorite childhood meals that my mom would make for us when we were young. It combines roasted eggplant, red peppers and mozzarella for a lunch that is both succulent and satisfying.

INGREDIENTS:

- 4 slices eggplant
- 2 ready-to-serve, grilled, boneless, skinless chicken breasts
- 2 thin or flatbread style sandwich rolls
- 1 jar red, roasted red pepper, sliced thinly
- JAT freshly ground black pepper
- 2 slices part-skim mozzarella cheese
- ⅔ cup baby spinach leaves

DIRECTIONS:

1. Preheat the broiler to high. Lightly coat a baking sheet with nonstick cooking spray. Arrange eggplant slices on the prepared sheet; broil for 3 minutes, turn and broil for an additional 3 minutes or until tender.

2. Warm the chicken breasts according to package directions. Top the sandwich roll bases with the chicken, eggplant, roasted pepper and black pepper. Top with mozzarella cheese. Place back under the broiler, just until the cheese melts. Top with the spinach and cap with the tops of the rolls. Serves 2.

JNL'S FUN, FIT FOODIE TIP:

Eggplant is a powerhouse veggie. Thanks to its high fiber content, it has been shown to help manage type 2 diabetes. It's an excellent source of vitamins B1, B6, and potassium, as well as a good source of copper, magnesium, manganese, phosphorus, niacin, and folic acid. Don't forget to eat the skin, as it's full of potent antioxidants that act as a free-radical scavenger.

NUTRIENTS PER SERVING
(1 sandwich)

Calories: 320	
Total Fat: 7g	
Saturated Fat: 3g	
Cholesterol: 75mg	
Sodium: 660mg	
Total Carbohydrate: 28g	
Dietary Fiber: 8g	
Sugars: 7g	
Protein: 39g	

% Daily Value
Vit A: 8%   Vit C: 50%
Calcium: 30%   Iron: 15%

Curried Turkey Burgers with Mango Chutney

My husband was born and raised in Jamaica, so I learned how to "curry in a hurry." I married into a strong culture with deep roots in their truly outstanding seasonings and ways of preparing their foods. I visit Jamaica often, and created this Fun, Fit Foodie recipe out of my love for all things curry and Caribbean!

INGREDIENTS:

- 1 ⅓ lb ground turkey breast
- 2 tbsp chopped fresh parsley
- 2 tbsp chopped fresh cilantro (optional)
- 2 scallions, thinly sliced
- 1 tbsp curry powder or paste
- 1-inch piece fresh ginger, grated or minced
- 2 cloves garlic, minced
- ½ red bell pepper, finely chopped
- 6 whole wheat hamburger or sandwich rolls
- Sweet mango chutney (such as Major Grey)
- Leaf lettuce, sliced tomatoes, sliced avocado (optional)

DIRECTIONS:

1. Mix the turkey with the parsley, cilantro (if using), scallions, curry powder, ginger, garlic and bell pepper until combined; shape into 6 equal size patties.

2. Preheat an indoor or outdoor grill to medium heat. Cook the patties, turning once, for 12 to 16 minutes or until cooked through. Serve on buns and garnish with chutney and other suggested toppings (if using) to taste. Serves 6.

NUTRIENTS PER SERVING
(1 burger with bun)

Calories: 420

Total Fat: 15g	
Saturated Fat: 3.5g	
Cholesterol: 75mg	
Sodium: 410mg	
Total Carbohydrate: 43g	
Dietary Fiber: 3g	
Sugars: 9g	
Protein: 29g	

% Daily Value
Vit A: 0%   Vit C: 50%
Calcium: 15%   Iron: 25%
Excellent source of thiamin, riboflavin, niacin, folate and selenium.

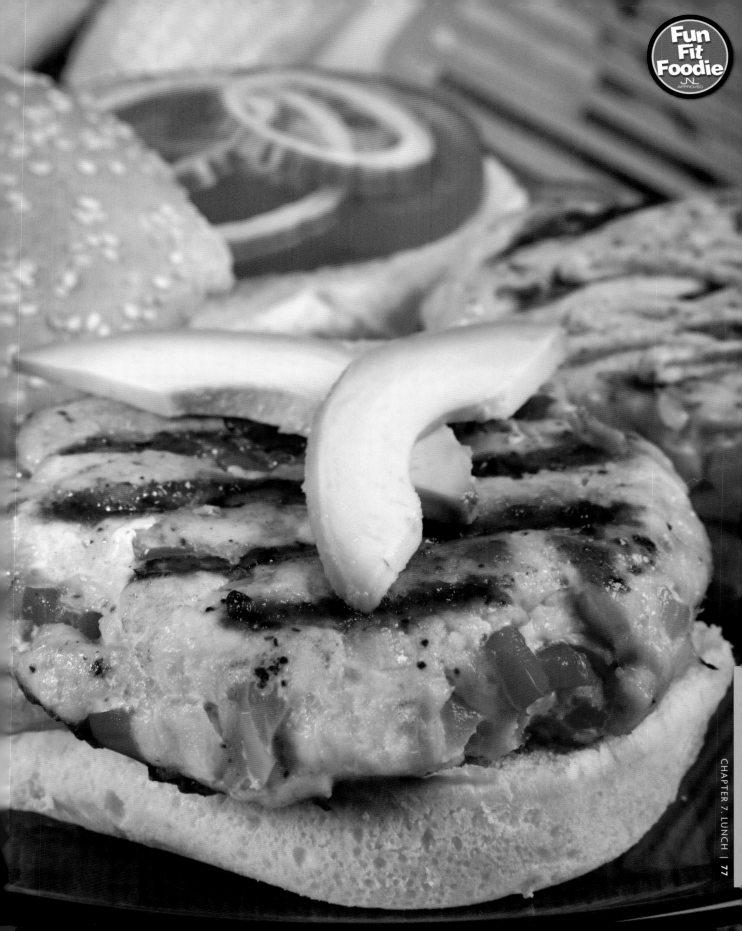

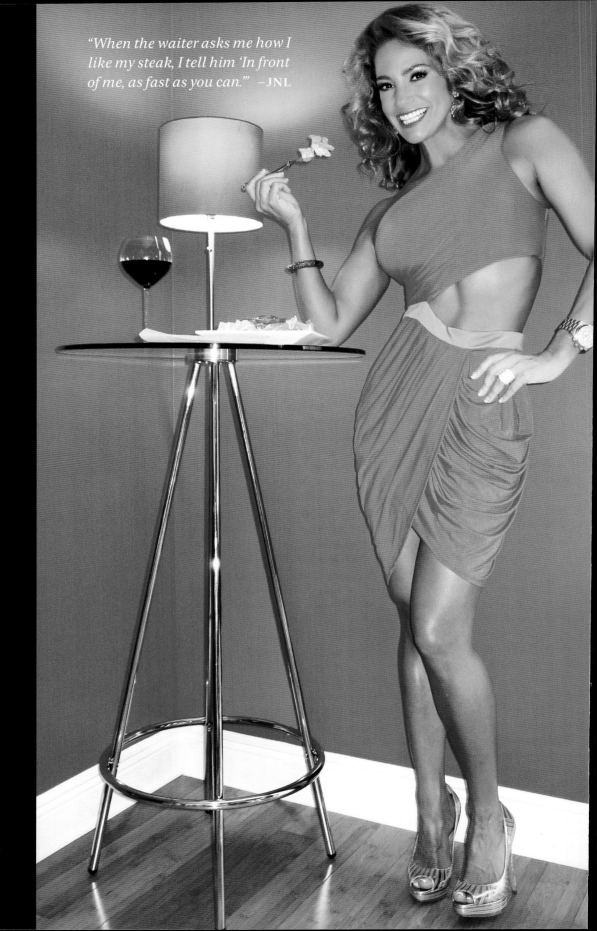

"When the waiter asks me how I like my steak, I tell him 'In front of me, as fast as you can.'" —JNL

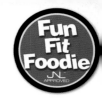

Diodato Eggplant Parmesan

This is one family recipe that my mom and I had to work out and perfect on our own, as her father never had a written version of it. It was one of the staples that he served in his Italian seaside restaurant in New York. He actually made it for me the one time that I met him, when I was around 8 years old. I went to visit, and he served up this massive meal with great pride and joy. I hope it warms your belly and spirit as it does mine. It's an original you will love! Serve with a crisp green salad for a complete meal.

INGREDIENTS:

- 1 whole egg
- 1 egg white
- 3 eggplants, peeled and thinly sliced
- 2 cups Italian seasoned breadcrumbs (approx.)
- 4 cups puréed fresh tomatoes (about 6 medium to large tomatoes)
- 16 oz part-skim mozzarella cheese, shredded and divided
- ½ cup grated light Parmesan cheese, divided
- ½ tsp dried basil
- ½ tsp Mrs. Dash Italian seasoning

DIRECTIONS:

1. Preheat oven to 350°F. Beat egg and egg white until combined. Dip eggplant slices in beaten egg, then in breadcrumbs. (Discard excess egg and crumbs). Place in a single layer on a baking sheet. Bake for 5 minutes per side.

2. Spread half of the pureed tomatoes into a 9x13-inch baking dish. Arrange half of the eggplant slices on top. Sprinkle with half of the mozzarella and Parmesan cheeses. Repeat layers once, ending with the cheeses. Sprinkle basil and seasoning evenly over the cheese.

3. Bake for 35 minutes, or until golden brown. Let stand for about 15 minutes to settle before serving. Serves 8.

NUTRIENTS PER SERVING

Calories: 320

Total Fat: 13g	
Saturated Fat: 7g	
Cholesterol: 60mg	
Sodium: 760mg	
Total Carbohydrate: 33g	
Dietary Fiber: 8g	
Sugars: 9g	
Protein: 22g	

% Daily Value
Vit A: 8%   Vit C: 25%
Calcium: 45%   Iron: 10%

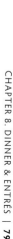

Baked Blackened Salmon Steaks with Mango and Black Bean Salsa

Salmon is my favorite fish; it's loaded with omega-3 fatty acids, which is great for our skin and fights off cancer. The only way to get essential omega-3 is through your food because your body does not make them. The fruit in the salsa adds a kick of sweetness and vitamin C. The black beans add fiber and are rich in antioxidants.

INGREDIENTS:

- 15 oz canned black beans, drained and rinsed
- 1 ½ cups diced mango (about 1 large)
- ½ cup diced kiwi
- ⅓ cup chopped cilantro
- 2 scallions, sliced
- 2 tsp honey
- ¼ tsp cayenne pepper
- JAT sea salt (optional)
- 1 lime, halved
- 4 salmon steaks (4 oz each)
- 2 tbsp salt-free blackening seasoning

DIRECTIONS:

1. Preheat the oven to 350°F. Toss the black beans with the mango, kiwi, cilantro, scallions, honey, cayenne pepper and sea salt (if using). Juice half of the lime over the mixture; toss to combine. Set aside.

2. Place salmon steaks on a baking dish. Drizzle the remaining lime juice over the fish. Sprinkle both sides with the blackening seasoning. Bake for 15 to 20 minutes or until cooked through. Serve each salmon steak on a bed of salsa. Serves 4.

NUTRIENTS PER SERVING

Calories: 380

Total Fat: 11g	
Saturated Fat: 1.5g	
Cholesterol: 80mg	
Sodium: 500mg	
Total Carbohydrate: 35g	
Dietary Fiber: 10g	
Sugars: 15g	
Protein: 37g	

% Daily Value
Vit A: 45%   Vit C: 120%
Calcium: 15%   Iron: 25%
Excellent source of folate, niacin, riboflavin, thiamin, vitamin B6, vitamin B12, vitamin D, magnesium and selenium.

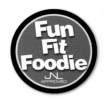

Chicken Broccoli Salad with Dried Cranberry & Sunflower Kernels

Save this Fun, Fit Foodie "recipe" for when you need a complete dinner in a flash! I love this recipe, as it's a healthy and tasty alternative to lettuce-based salads. You can use leftover cooked chicken or a can of all-white chunk chicken if you are in a pinch. The salad is all ready to go; simply open the bag and mix. It contains shredded broccoli, carrots, red cabbage, and broccoli florets, as well as soy nuts, sunflower kernels, dried cranberries and a zesty dressing.

INGREDIENTS:

- 1 bag (12 oz) Eat Smart Broccoli Salad Kit
- 1 cup chopped, cooked, boneless skinless chicken breast
- Chopped, toasted walnuts (optional)

DIRECTIONS:

1. Prepare the salad kit according to package directions. Simply toss in the chicken. Sprinkle with walnuts (if using). Serves 2.

NUTRIENTS PER SERVING

Calories: 290
Total Fat: 9g
Saturated Fat: 0g
Cholesterol: 60mg
Sodium: 270mg
Total Carbohydrate: 20g
Dietary Fiber: 6g
Sugars: 10g
Protein: 31g

% Daily Value
Vit A: 30%   Vit C: 200%
Calcium: 8%   Iron: 10%

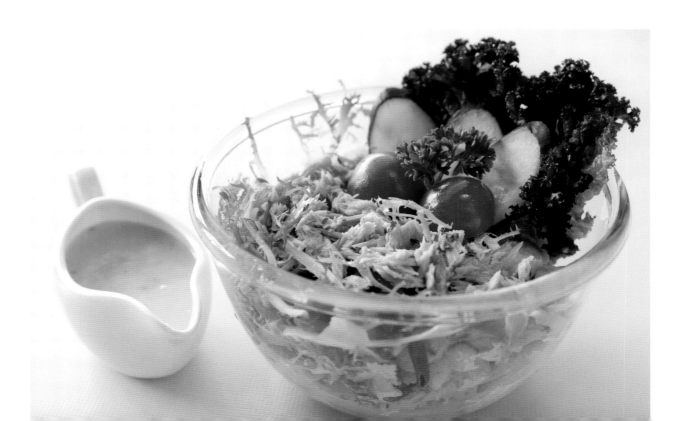

Ocean Drive Paella

There is nothing like strolling down the famous Ocean Drive on South Beach and stopping for a delicious plate of fresh seafood paella, served at a table overlooking the ocean. Even if you are far from the seashore, that doesn't mean you can't enjoy this super flavorful meal. To bring this experience into your home, simply follow my recipe for a healthier version.

INGREDIENTS:

- 1 cup long-grain brown rice
- 2 cups low sodium vegetable broth
- 1 tbsp olive oil, divided
- 1 link (4 oz) turkey kielbasa, sliced
- 4 (4 oz each) skinless, boneless chicken breasts, cut into bite-size pieces
- 12 large raw shrimp, peeled and de-veined
- 12 mussels (about ½ lb)
- 18 littleneck clams
- 1 each medium-sized red, green and yellow pepper, chopped

- 1 cup chopped red onion
- 1 cup asparagus tips
- ½ cup sliced button mushrooms
- ½ cup fresh or frozen green peas
- 2 cloves garlic, minced
- 1 ½ cups chopped tomato
- ¼ cup finely chopped fresh flat-leaf parsley, divided
- ½ tsp turmeric

DIRECTIONS:

1. Combine the rice and broth in a large saucepan; set over high heat and bring to a boil. Cover, reduce the heat to low and simmer rice for 40 minutes.

2. Meanwhile, heat half of the oil in a large skillet set over medium heat, until hot but not smoking. Add the kielbasa. Cook until browned all over; transfer to a plate. Add the chicken to the skillet and cook, stirring, for 4 minutes or until browned. Transfer to the plate with the sausage. Repeat the same process with the shrimp, cooking until pink.

3. Place a steamer over a pot of boiling water. Add the clams and mussels; cover and steam for 15 minutes. Discard any unopened shells.

4. Preheat the oven to 400°F. Heat the remaining oil in the skillet. Add the peppers, onion, asparagus, mushrooms, peas and garlic. Sauté for about 5 minutes or until the asparagus is just barely tender. Stir in the tomatoes, cooked rice, half of the parsley and the turmeric until combined.

5. Transfer to an ovenproof serving dish. Arrange the chicken, shrimp, clams and mussels on top, nestling into the rice. Bake, uncovered, for about 10 minutes or until warmed through. Cover tightly with aluminum foil and let stand 15 minutes. Sprinkle with the remaining parsley and serve immediately. Serves 6.

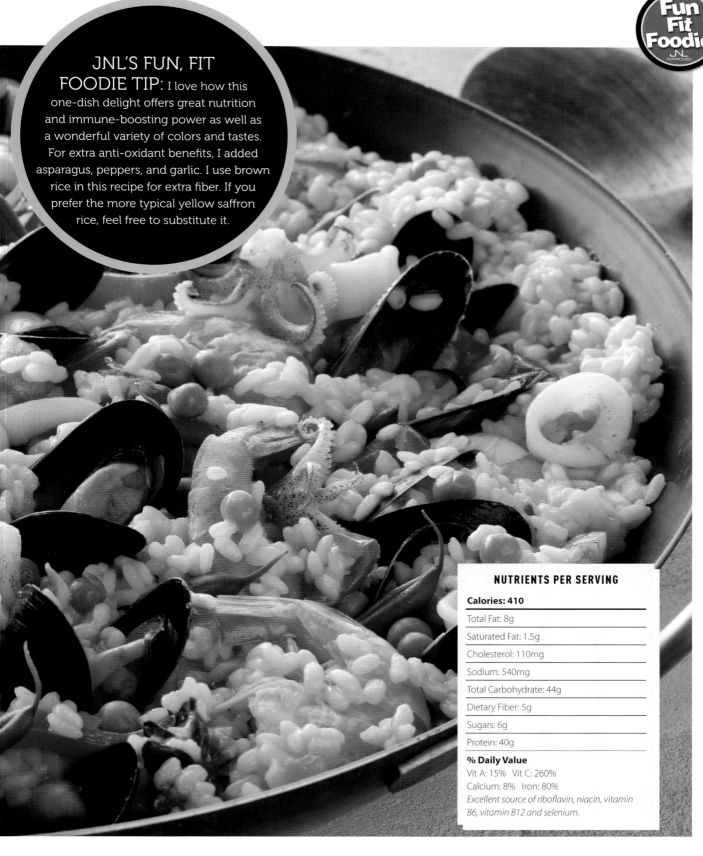

JNL'S FUN, FIT FOODIE TIP: I love how this one-dish delight offers great nutrition and immune-boosting power as well as a wonderful variety of colors and tastes. For extra anti-oxidant benefits, I added asparagus, peppers, and garlic. I use brown rice in this recipe for extra fiber. If you prefer the more typical yellow saffron rice, feel free to substitute it.

NUTRIENTS PER SERVING

Calories: 410

Total Fat: 8g

Saturated Fat: 1.5g

Cholesterol: 110mg

Sodium: 540mg

Total Carbohydrate: 44g

Dietary Fiber: 5g

Sugars: 6g

Protein: 40g

% Daily Value
Vit A: 15%   Vit C: 260%
Calcium: 8%   Iron: 80%
Excellent source of riboflavin, niacin, vitamin B6, vitamin B12 and selenium.

Spicy Tilapia Tacos with Crispy Veggie & Corn Salsa

WOW! What a kick this fish has! Light, flaky, meatier than most, and not fishy smelling at all. The spicy fish fillets are offset with the cool, crisp salsa made up of crunchy fresh corn. I like to prepare this when my fitness friends come over, or for my hubby on Saturdays pool-side, while our sons are playing outside.

INGREDIENTS:

- 1 cup corn
- 1 cup lightly packed fresh cilantro leaves, finely chopped
- ¾ cup mixed diced red, yellow and green bell peppers
- ½ cup diced white onion
- 1 lime, juiced
- 2 tbsp cayenne pepper
- 1 tbsp ground black pepper
- 6 (4 oz) tilapia fillets
- 2 tbsp canola oil
- 12 small whole wheat or spinach tortillas, warmed
- 1 avocado, diced or HOLY MOLY Guacamole *(see recipe page 121)*
- 2 tbsp fat-free sour cream

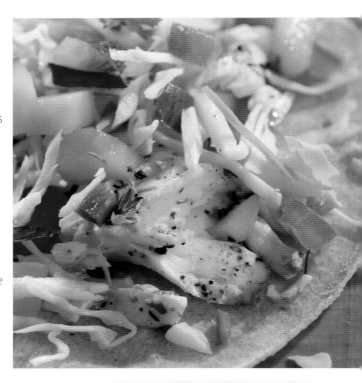

DIRECTIONS:

1. Toss corn with cilantro, peppers, onion and lime juice. Set aside.

2. Preheat the grill or a lightly greased heavy skillet to high. Toss cayenne with black pepper in a shallow bowl. Lightly coat each piece of fish with oil and then dip one side into the spice blend. Grill fish for 3 minutes per side.

3. Flake fish into chunks and divide between tortillas. Top with salsa, sour cream and avocado. Serves 6.

NUTRIENTS PER SERVING
(2 tacos)

Calories: 450	
Total Fat: 19g	
Saturated Fat: 2g	
Cholesterol: 65mg	
Sodium: 500mg	
Total Carbohydrate: 40g	
Dietary Fiber: 8g	
Sugars: 2g	
Protein: 32g	

% Daily Value
Vit A: 2%   Vit C: 60%
Calcium: 8%   Iron: 4%

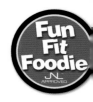

Indian-Style Beef Kabobs with "Snappy" Bulgur

The marinade for this dish is made with molasses, which is excellent for the man in your life, as it helps to reduce the size of the prostate. Bulgur is man's oldest recorded use of wheat. Bulgur is convenient, since it can be either soaked in water or cooked to be edible with the same nutritive value as whole-grain wheat. The bulgur here is called "snappy" because it's got a sweet and spicy kick to it, and it also whips up in a snap!

INGREDIENTS:

- 1 lb boneless beef tenderloin steaks, about 1-inch thick
- ¼ cup un-sulphured molasses
- 3 tbsp fresh squeezed orange juice
- 2 cloves garlic, minced
- ¼ tsp ground cumin

"Snappy" Bulgur:

- ½ cup uncooked quick-cooking bulgur
- ½ cup water
- ¾ cup diced dried apricots
- ¼ cup fresh squeezed orange juice
- ½ tsp pumpkin pie spice
- ½ tsp ground cumin
- 1 clove garlic, minced
- 2 tbsp chopped fresh parsley

DIRECTIONS:

1. Cut the beef into 1 ¼-inch cubes. Whisk molasses with orange juice, garlic and cumin until well mixed; add the beef cubes to the bowl (making sure all the cubes are covered). Marinate in the fridge for at least 30 minutes or up to 2 hours.

2. "Snappy" Bulgur: Meanwhile, combine the bulgur, water, apricots, juice, pumpkin pie spice, cumin, and garlic in small saucepan; bring to a rapid boil. Reduce the heat to low; cover and simmer for 15 minutes or until bulgur is cooked all the way through but not mushy. Fluff with a fork. Add the parsley and toss to combine.

3. Meanwhile, preheat the grill to medium-high. Remove beef from marinade (discard marinade). Thread the beef cubes onto pre-soaked bamboo or metal skewers, leaving a small space between cubes. Place the kabobs on the grill; cook, turning as needed until cooked to your preferred doneness. Serve over the warm bulgur. Serves 4.

NUTRIENTS PER SERVING

Calories: 330

Total Fat: 7g	
Saturated Fat: 2.5g	
Cholesterol: 70mg	
Sodium: 70mg	
Total Carbohydrate: 35g	
Dietary Fiber: 4g	
Sugars: 18g	
Protein: 31g	

% Daily Value
Vit A: 0%   Vit C: 20%
Calcium: 6%   Iron: 20%
Excellent source of niacin, vitamin B6, vitamin B12, selenium and zinc.

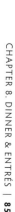

Savory Asian Beef

I'm an ambassador for heart health, so I'm happy to be sharing some of my all-time favorite recipes that will help you to avoid heart disease, the #1 killer for women. This is a great recipe adapted from the American Heart Association's *Go Red™ for Women Cookbook*. May your heart enjoy its healthy benefits!

INGREDIENTS:

- 1 scallion, finely chopped
- 2 garlic cloves, minced
- 1 ½ tbsp dry sherry
- 1 tbsp oyster sauce
- 1 ½ tsp hoisin sauce
- 1 ½ tsp toasted sesame oil
- ½ tsp grated fresh ginger root
- ½ tsp no-salt-added liquid smoke flavorings
- ¼ tsp granulated sugar (or honey)
- JAT fresh ground pepper
- JAT hot pepper sauce
- 1 lb boneless sirloin steak, all visible fat discarded, cut across the grain into strips

JNL FUN, FIT FOODIE TIP: Serve this flavorful beef over brown rice with lots of stir-fried vegetables on the side. Stir-frying is an excellent way to combine a lean source of protein, antioxidant-rich vegetables, and high-fiber carbs (when you serve your stir-fry with brown rice). Loading up on veggies and rice may also cut your diabetes risk. It's been found that enjoying a veggie-packed diet decreases insulin resistance. In addition, studies suggest that those who consume a cup or more of brown rice every 7 to 10 days have over a 13% lower chance of developing diabetes. Need another reason to enjoy brown rice and vegetables? The antioxidants in whole grains and vegetables prevent cell damage.

DIRECTIONS:

1. Stir the scallion, garlic, sherry, oyster sauce, hoisin, sesame oil, ginger, liquid smoke, sugar, pepper and hot sauce in a large glass dish. Add the steak, turning to coat. Cover and place in the fridge for about 1 hour, turning every 15 minutes. Drain, discarding the marinade.

2. Coat a large skillet with nonstick cooking spray; set over medium heat until hot. Add the steak in a single layer (in batches as needed). Cook for about 1 to 2 minutes per each side. (Turn only once, or the meat will become dry and tough.) Serves 4.

NUTRIENTS PER SERVING
(steak only)

Calories: 160	
Total Fat: 5g	
Saturated Fat: 1.5g	
Cholesterol: 65mg	
Sodium: 100mg	
Total Carbohydrate: 1g	
Dietary Fiber: 0g	
Sugars: 0g	
Protein: 27g	

% Daily Value
Vit A: 0%   Vit C: 0%
Calcium: 0%   Iron: 15%
Excellent source of niacin and vitamin B12

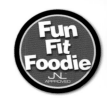

Indian Style Lamb Shanks

A Fun, Fit Foodie dish that will delight all at dinner. Preparing lamb shank typically requires a long cooking time to tenderize the meat. Using a pressure cooker allows you to make this tasty meal in a snap! Serve with steamed, seasonal vegetables.

INGREDIENTS:

- 4 lamb shanks (about 1 lb each)
- JAT fresh ground black pepper
- 1 sweet potato, peeled and cut into bite-size chunks
- 2 tbsp extra virgin olive oil
- 1 can (14.5 oz) no salt added, petite diced tomatoes
- ½ cup red wine
- ½ cup low sodium chicken broth
- 2 tbsp tomatoes paste
- 1 shallot, minced
- 3 cloves garlic, minced
- ½ tsp each cumin and coriander seeds
- ½ tsp pumpkin pie spice
- ½ tsp grated fresh ginger
- 1 (½-inch length) cinnamon stick
- 2 tbsp chopped fresh cilantro

DIRECTIONS:

1. Season the lamb shanks with pepper and arrange in the pressure cooker. Scatter the sweet potatoes around the shanks. Drizzle with olive oil.

2. Stir tomatoes with the red wine, chicken broth, tomato paste, shallot, garlic, cumin, coriander, pumpkin pie spice, ginger and the cinnamon stick; add to the pressure cooker. Set the pressure cooker to cook for 20 minutes. Check, if the meat isn't tender, set the pressure cooker for an additional 10 minutes. Discard cinnamon stick and garnish with cilantro. Serves 4.

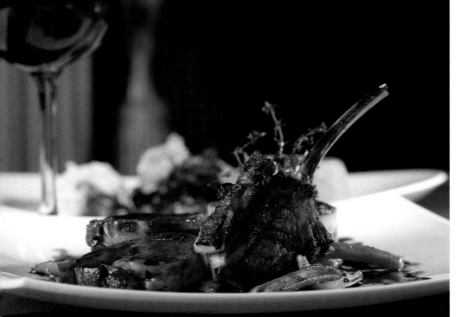

NUTRIENTS PER SERVING

Calories: 370

Total Fat: 13g	
Saturated Fat: 3g	
Cholesterol: 105mg	
Sodium: 230mg	
Total Carbohydrate: 23g	
Dietary Fiber: 4g	
Sugars: 7g	
Protein: 34g	

% Daily Value
Vit A: 40%   Vit C: 15%
Calcium: 15%   Iron: 20%
Excellent source of niacin, vitamin B12, manganese, selenium and zinc.

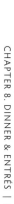

Chicken in Red Wine Sauce

Another great recipe adapted from the American Heart Association's cookbook! By replacing regular pork bacon with turkey bacon, you still get a ton of flavor, without the ton of fat.

INGREDIENTS:

- 2 slices turkey bacon, chopped
- 12 small button mushrooms
- 12 pearl onions or small shallots
- 2 garlic cloves, minced
- 1 cup full-bodied red wine
- 1 cup low sodium chicken broth
- 1 tbsp no salt added tomato paste
- ½ tsp crumbled dried oregano
- ½ tsp dried thyme
- 1 bay leaf
- 1 ½ lb boneless, skinless chicken breasts
- 2 tbsp all-purpose flour
- JAT fresh ground pepper

DIRECTIONS:

1. Cook the bacon, stirring occasionally in a large skillet or Dutch oven set over medium heat for 5 minutes or until browned. Stir in the mushrooms, onions, and garlic. Cook, stirring occasionally, for 5 minutes. Meanwhile, in a small bowl, stir together the wine, broth, tomato paste, oregano, thyme, and bay leaf.

2. Add the chicken to the skillet. Pour the wine mixture over the chicken. Increase the heat to high and bring to a boil. Reduce the heat to low and simmer, covered, for 25 minutes, or until chicken is tender and no longer pink in the center. Use a slotted spoon to transfer the chicken to a plate, tent with foil to keep warm. Discard the bay leaf.

3. In a small bowl, whisk the flour with about ¼ cup of the liquid from the skillet until smooth. Whisk back into skillet. Increase the heat to medium. Cook, stirring often, for 5 to 10 minutes, or until thickened and bubbly. Season with pepper. Return the chicken to the skillet. Reduce the heat to low and cook, covered for 5 minutes or until warmed through. Remove from the heat and let stand for 2 minutes. Serves 6.

NUTRIENTS PER SERVING

Calories: 200

Total Fat: 3g	
Saturated Fat: 1g	
Cholesterol: 75mg	
Sodium: 250mg	
Total Carbohydrate: 6g	
Dietary Fiber: 1g	
Sugars: 2g	
Protein: 30g	

% Daily Value
Vit A: 2%   Vit C: 4%
Calcium: 2%   Iron: 6%
Excellent source of niacin, vitamin B6, selenium.

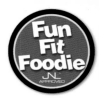

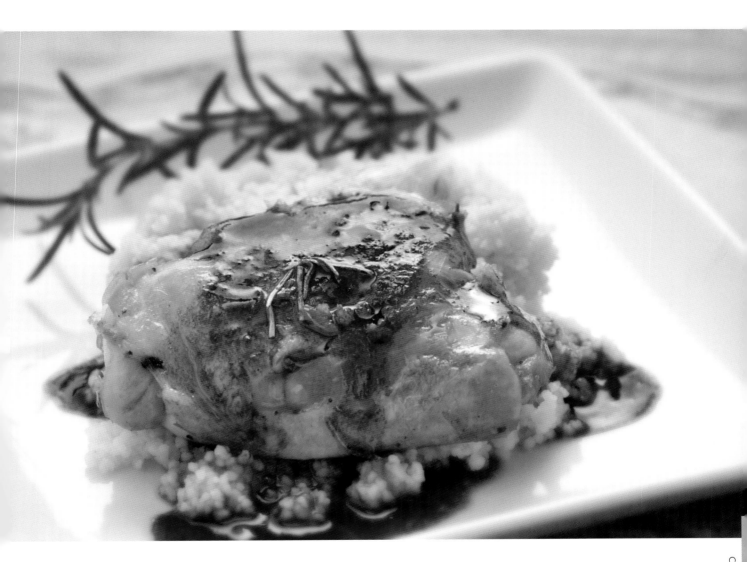

CHAPTER 8: DINNER & ENTRÉS | **89**

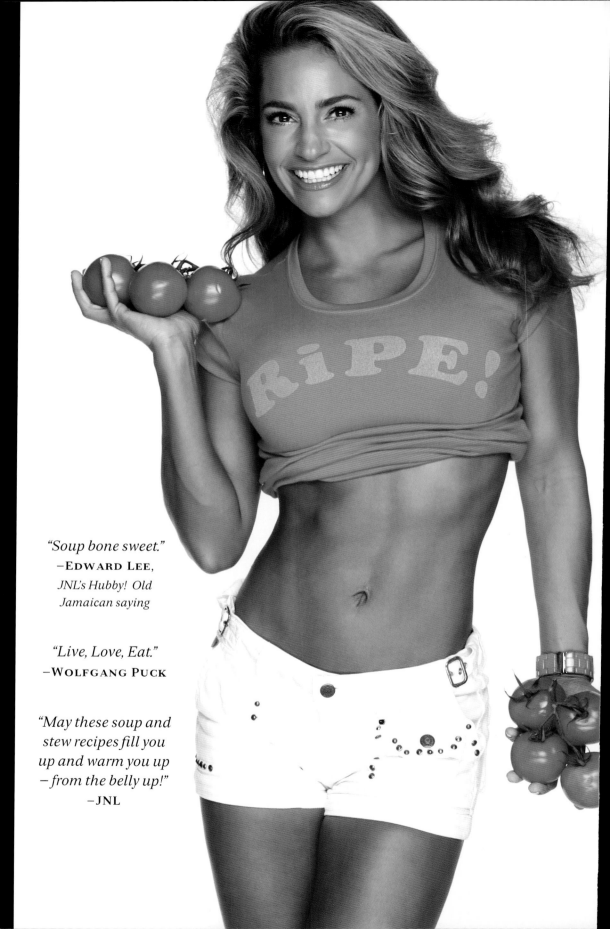

9. SOUPS & STEWS

"Soup bone sweet."
—EDWARD LEE,
JNL's Hubby! Old Jamaican saying

"Live, Love, Eat."
—WOLFGANG PUCK

"May these soup and stew recipes fill you up and warm you up – from the belly up!"
—JNL

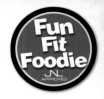

JNL's Birthday Minestrone Soup

This recipe is near and dear to my heart, as it is what my Italian-born grandfather, Nicholas Diodato, cooked for our entire family in celebration of my birth and the fact that I was named after him. Nicholas prided himself on cooking hearty meals that warmed you from the belly up. I'm honored to share my rendition of this classic, in honor of my mom's dad. Here it's shown as a vegetarian version. For a meaty soup, add 2 cups lean (4 % fat) cooked ground beef.

INGREDIENTS:

- 3 cups low sodium vegetable or chicken broth
- 1 can (15-oz) white cannellini beans, drained and rinsed
- ½ cup full bodied red wine such as Cabernet Sauvignon
- 3 Roma tomatoes, diced
- 2 carrots, peeled and chopped
- 1 celery stalk, chopped
- 1 cup white onion, chopped
- 1 tsp dried thyme
- ½ tsp dried sage
- 2 bay leaves
- JAT each sea salt and fresh ground black pepper
- ¾ cup dry ditalini or another soup-style pasta cut
- 1 medium zucchini, chopped
- 2 cups coarsely chopped fresh spinach
- 1 oz chunk of good quality Parmesan cheese (such as Parmigiana Reggiano)
- Fresh basil leaves (optional)

> **JNL'S FUN, FIT FOODIE TIP:** The small chunk of Parmesan cheese will "melt" into the soups broth, and thicken it, by adding a distinct, yet delicate, authentic Italian flavor.

DIRECTIONS:

1. In a slow cooker, combine broth, beans, wine, tomatoes, carrots, celery, onion, thyme, sage, bay leaves, salt and black pepper. Cook on the LOW setting for about 6 hours or on the HIGH setting for about 3 hours.

2. Add ditalini, zucchini, spinach and cheese. Cover and cook on HIGH for 30 additional minutes. Discard bay leaves and season to taste with additional salt and black pepper. Garnish with basil leaves (if using). Serves 4.

NUTRIENTS PER SERVING

Calories: 290

Total Fat: 2.5g	
Saturated Fat: 1.5g	
Cholesterol: 5mg	
Sodium: 690mg	
Total Carbohydrate: 48g	
Dietary Fiber: 8g	
Sugars: 8g	
Protein: 16g	

% Daily Value
Vit A: 2%   Vit C: 40%
Calcium: 20%   Iron: 20%
Excellent source of folate and selenium.

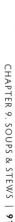

JNL Coconut Thai Chicken Soup

It's been proven that soup fills you up quickly, thus curbing your appetite. This is a great soup to have if you feel a cold coming on. The hot pepper helps to fight off fever and the coconut oil boosts your immune system. This soup is a great addition to a healthy food plan.

INGREDIENTS:

- 1 tbsp canola oil
- 1 tsp coconut oil
- 1 cup red bell pepper, sliced lengthwise
- 1 cup broccoli
- 4 shallots, chopped
- 2 small fresh red chili peppers, chopped
- 1 clove garlic, chopped
- 1 tbsp chopped lemongrass
- 2 ⅛ cups low sodium chicken broth
- 1 ½ cups unsweetened light (or lite) coconut milk
- 6 oz boneless, skinless chicken breast, cut into bite-size chunks
- JAT cayenne pepper
- 1 small bunch fresh basil leaves, coarsely chopped

DIRECTIONS:

1. Heat the canola and coconut oils in a saucepan set over medium-low heat. Add the red pepper, broccoli, shallots, chili peppers, garlic and lemongrass; cook, stirring, for 2 to 3 minutes or until fragrant.

2. Stir in the chicken broth, coconut milk and chicken; bring to a simmer. Simmer on low heat until chicken is cooked. Add cayenne pepper (to taste). Stir in the basil just before serving. Serves 4.

JNL'S FUN, FIT FOODIE TIP:

Make any soup in double or triple batches; cool and freeze into individual portions. Warm it up in the microwave for a hot, delicious snack that will fill you up without filling you with guilt!

NUTRIENTS PER SERVING

Calories: 180

Total Fat: 8g	
Saturated Fat: 6g	
Cholesterol: 25mg	
Sodium: 200mg	
Total Carbohydrate: 13g	
Dietary Fiber: 3g	
Sugars: 5g	
Protein: 13g	

% Daily Value
Vit A: 2%   Vit C: 210%
Calcium: 6%   Iron: 15%
Excellent source of niacin and vitamin B6.

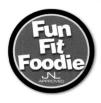

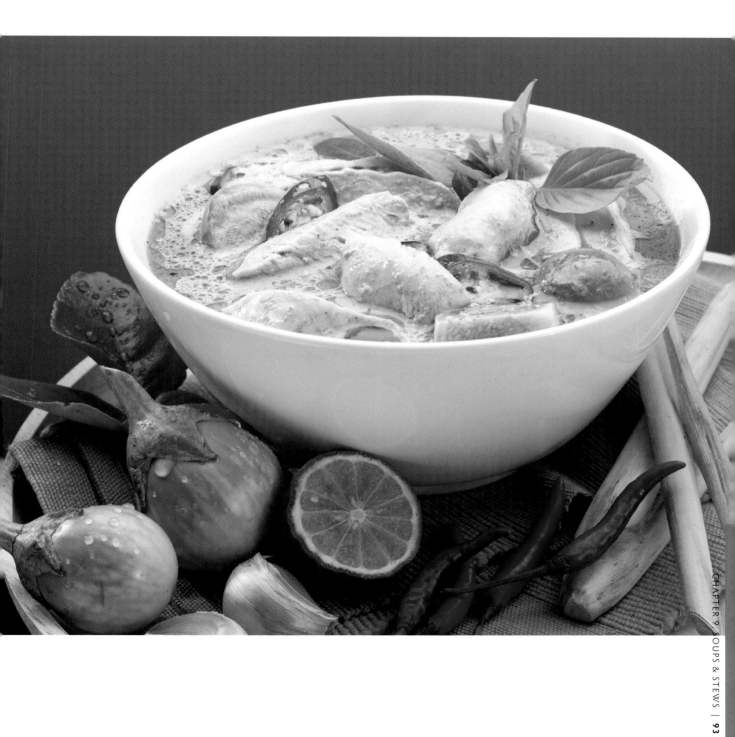

Game Day Chili

When it's cold outside, and the game is on, and you've got a bunch of hungry, raving sports fans to feed, lean on this hearty chili recipe! By substituting half of the ground beef that is called for in the original recipe with lean ground turkey, you cut out tons of fat and unnecessary empty calories. Top with fresh chopped tomatoes, scallion, and a dollop of fat-free sour cream and you've got a dish that will make 'em holler "touchdown"!

INGREDIENTS:

- ½ lb each extra lean ground beef
- ½ lb extra lean ground turkey
- ½ cup each dried pinto beans, black beans and red kidney beans, rinsed and picked over
- ½ cup pearl barley
- 2 large onions, finely chopped
- 2 carrots, finely chopped
- 2 stalks celery, finely chopped
- 2 jalapeño peppers, seeded and chopped
- 1 can (4 oz) chopped green chilies, drained
- 6 cloves garlic, minced
- 1 tbsp chili powder
- 2 tsp ground cumin
- 1 tsp dried oregano
- 1 bay leaf
- 6 cups water
- 1 cup low sodium vegetable or chicken broth
- 1 can(28 oz) plum tomatoes, drained and chopped
- JAT Freshly ground black pepper
- Fat free sour cream, chopped tomatoes and chopped scallion (optional)

DIRECTIONS

1. Stir the beef, turkey, dried beans, barley, onions, carrots, celery, jalapeño peppers, chilies, garlic, chili powder, cumin, oregano and bay leaf together in a pressure cooker until combined. Add the water, plum tomatoes and broth. Stir to combine.

2. Set the pressure cooker for 20 minutes. Check the beans, if still too firm, set the pressure cooker for 10 additional minutes. Season with pepper. Garnish with sour cream, tomatoes and scallion (if using). Makes 6 servings.

NUTRIENTS PER SERVING

Calories: 400

Total Fat: 6g	
Saturated Fat: 2g	
Cholesterol: 55mg	
Sodium: 440mg	
Total Carbohydrate: 57g	
Dietary Fiber: 12g	
Sugars: 8g	
Protein: 29g	

% Daily Value
Vit A: 15%   Vit C: 50%
Calcium: 15%   Iron: 35%
Excellent source of thiamin, vitamin B6, folate, magnesium, selenium and zinc.

JNL'S FUN, FIT FOODIE TIP: Several of my Fun, Fit Foodie friends are vegetarians, and my husband is a real meat-and-potatoes kind of guy. So this recipe fits perfectly in my meal arsenal, as I can add or take out the meat, to make everyone happy!

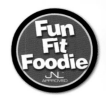

Pulled Chicken Baked Beans

Yes, you probably think of this as a side dish more commonly made with pulled pork, but I have given this comfort food a Fun, Fit Foodie make over. Just replace the pork with boneless, skinless chicken breast, and you have a hearty, stick-to-your-ribs, good meal, much too substantial to be called a side dish.

INGREDIENTS:

- 7 ½ cups water
- 1 cup apple cider
- ½ cup drained, canned chopped tomatoes
- ⅓ cup un-sulphured molasses
- ¼ cup firmly packed dark brown sugar
- 1 tsp dry mustard powder
- 1 bay leaf
- 2 boneless, skinless chicken breasts
- 1 cup dry navy or great northern beans, rinsed and picked over
- 1 cup chopped onion

DIRECTIONS:

1. Stir the water with the cider, tomatoes, molasses, brown sugar, mustard powder and bay leaf. Arrange the chicken, beans and onion in a pressure cooker. Pour over the cider mixture.

2. Set the pressure cooker for 20 minutes. Check the beans, if still too firm, set the pressure cooker for 10 additional minutes. Remove the chicken breasts to a bowl. Use two forks to pull the meat into shreds. Stir the chicken back into the beans to create a thick, rich, stew-like dish. Serves 6.

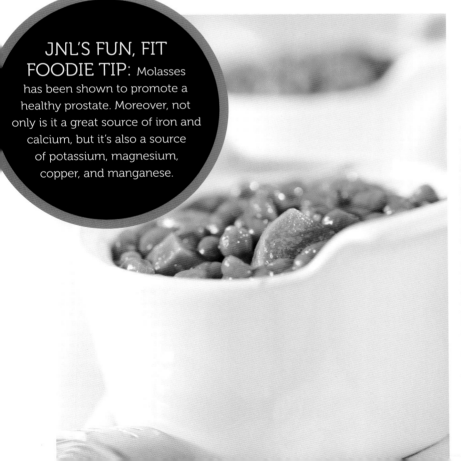

JNL'S FUN, FIT FOODIE TIP: Molasses has been shown to promote a healthy prostate. Moreover, not only is it a great source of iron and calcium, but it's also a source of potassium, magnesium, copper, and manganese.

NUTRIENTS PER SERVING

Calories: 350

Total Fat: 6g	
Saturated Fat: 1.5g	
Cholesterol: 35mg	
Sodium: 90mg	
Total Carbohydrate: 54g	
Dietary Fiber: 7g	
Sugars: 27g	
Protein: 21g	

% Daily Value
Vit A: 2%   Vit C: 25%
Calcium: 10%   Iron: 20%
Excellent source of thiamin, niacin, vitamin B6, folate, magnesium, manganese and selenium.

Texas Two Step Stew

This all-time favorite has gotten a Fun, Fit Foodie makeover, by replacing the full-fat sausage called for in the original recipe with turkey chorizo sausage. Feel free to use boneless, skinless chicken breasts instead, if you prefer.

INGREDIENTS:

- 8 oz uncooked turkey chorizo sausage, casings removed
- 1 medium onion, chopped
- 1 cup drained and rinsed, canned black beans
- 1 can (15 oz) hominy
- 1 pkg (6 oz) Spanish-style rice mix
- 6 cups water

DIRECTIONS:

1. Lightly coat a skillet with cooking spray; set over medium heat. Add the sausage with onion; cook, stirring, until sausage is no longer pink. Drain off any fat. Transfer the sausage mixture to a pressure cooker.

2. Add the beans, hominy, rice mix (including the seasoning packet). Pour in the water. Set the pressure cooker for 20 minutes. Serves 6.

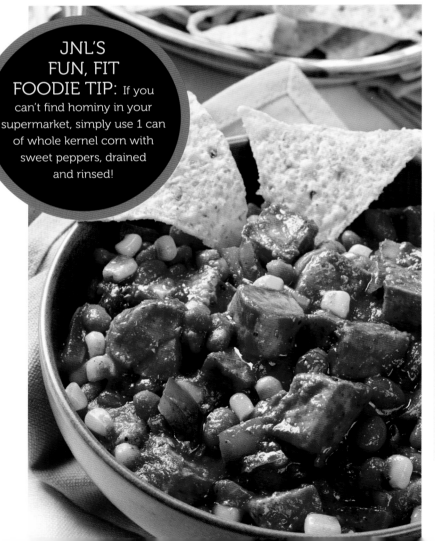

JNL'S FUN, FIT FOODIE TIP: If you can't find hominy in your supermarket, simply use 1 can of whole kernel corn with sweet peppers, drained and rinsed!

NUTRIENTS PER SERVING

Calories: 300

Total Fat: 2.5g	
Saturated Fat: 0g	
Cholesterol: 20mg	
Sodium: 890mg	
Total Carbohydrate: 54g	
Dietary Fiber: 9g	
Sugars: 4g	
Protein: 16g	

% Daily Value
Vit A: 20%   Vit C: 10%
Calcium: 10%   Iron: 25%
Excellent source of thiamin and folate.

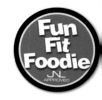

Red and Brown Lentils with Italian Turkey Sausage

Preparing this recipe is a CINCH! It's a complete meal in a bowl, packed full of protein and fiber, which will keep you full until the morning. Lentils are an excellent source of iron along with that protein and fiber, which will make your body feel like the powerhouse that it is, the Fun, Fit Foodie way!

INGREDIENTS:

- ½ lb sweet Italian turkey sausage, cut into 1-inch pieces
- 1 medium onion
- 1 large sweet potato, peeled and cut into bite-sized chunks (optional)
- 1 large carrot, peeled and cut into bite-sized chunks
- 1 stalk of celery, thinly sliced
- ½ cup dried red lentils
- ½ cup dried brown lentils
- 2 cups low sodium chicken broth
- 1 can (14.5 oz) diced tomatoes with garlic and olive oil flavor
- 1 bay leaf
- 1 tsp parsley paste
- 1 tsp garlic paste

> **JNL'S FUN, FIT FOODIE TIP:** I love my pressure cooker! All you have to do is place all the ingredients inside and push one button. Now, that's the kind of "cooking" I like! While my pressure cooker is doing its job, I can bang out my workout, and then sit down and enjoy my post-workout meal. This is the Fun, Fit Foodie lifestyle that I love, and so does my body.

DIRECTIONS:

1. Add sausage, onion, sweet potato (if using), carrot, celery, red and brown lentils to a pressure cooker. Stir in the broth, diced tomatoes, bay leaf, parsley and garlic pastes. Set the pressure cooker for 20 minutes. Stir well before serving. Serves 4.

NUTRIENTS PER SERVING

Calories: 260

Total Fat: 10g	
Saturated Fat: 2.5g	
Cholesterol: 25mg	
Sodium: 600mg	
Total Carbohydrate: 28g	
Dietary Fiber: 5g	
Sugars: 7g	
Protein: 15g	

% Daily Value
Vit A: 10%   Vit C: 15%
Calcium: 4%   Iron: 20%

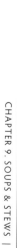

Spicy Winter Squash Soup

Squash is loaded with vitamin C (great for boosting your immune system and to fight off colds) and fiber (to keep your digestive system working regularly). The cayenne is great for circulation, and the coconut oil has medicinal properties to fight off infections and hyper-thyroidism. But your family won't even think of how good this soup is for them, because of how rich and delicious it is!

INGREDIENTS:

- 1 large winter squash (such as butternut or buttercup), halved and seeded
- 1 sweet potato, well scrubbed
- 1 medium Spanish onion
- 2 tsp virgin coconut oil
- 2 ½ tsp curry powder
- ½ tsp cayenne pepper
- JAT cinnamon
- JAT black pepper
- 4 cups low sodium chicken or vegetable broth
- Fat-free sour cream or yogurt
- Whole wheat croutons

DIRECTIONS:

1. Preheat the oven to 350°F. Arrange the squash and sweet potato on a baking sheet. Bake for 45 minutes or until soft. Scoop out the flesh of the squash and purée in a food processor until smooth. Peel and cube the sweet potato. Set aside.

2. In a large saucepan set over medium heat, sauté the onion in the coconut oil for 2 minutes. Add curry powder, cayenne pepper, cinnamon and pepper; stir to coat. Add the broth, squash and sweet potatoes; bring to a boil. Reduce heat to medium-low; cook, partially covered, for 7 to 10 minutes. Serve each portion with a dollop of sour cream and whole-wheat croutons. Serves 6.

NUTRIENTS PER SERVING

Calories: 130

Total Fat: 2g	
Saturated Fat: 1.5g	
Cholesterol: 0mg	
Sodium: 210mg	
Total Carbohydrate: 28g	
Dietary Fiber: 4g	
Sugars: 8g	
Protein: 4g	

% Daily Value
Vit A: 0%   Vit C: 70%
Calcium: 10%   Iron: 8%
Excellent source of manganese.

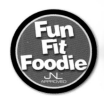

Pumpkin Curry Soup

Pumpkin isn't just for Halloween; loaded with beta-carotene and vitamin C to help boost your immune system. This flavorful soup comes together in a snap. Only, be sure to use 100% pure pumpkin and not pumpkin pie filling!

INGREDIENTS:

- 2 tbsp olive oil
- ½ cup chopped white onion
- 2 tsp curry powder
- JAT freshly ground black pepper
- 4 cups low sodium chicken broth or vegetable broth
- 1 can (15 oz) pure pumpkin purée
- 2 sweet potatoes, peeled and cut into 1-inch cubes
- ¼ cup chopped fresh cilantro
- Fat free sour cream (optional)
- Chives (optional)

DIRECTIONS:

1. Heat the oil in a large saucepan set over medium heat. Add the onion and cook until transparent. Stir in the curry powder and pepper.

2. Stir in the broth, pumpkin and sweet potatoes. Bring to a boil; cook for 1 minute. Reduce the heat to medium; simmer for 10 minutes, or until sweet potatoes are tender. Remove from the heat and stir in the cilantro. Garnish each bowl with a small dollop of sour cream and a sprinkle of chives (if using). Serves 4.

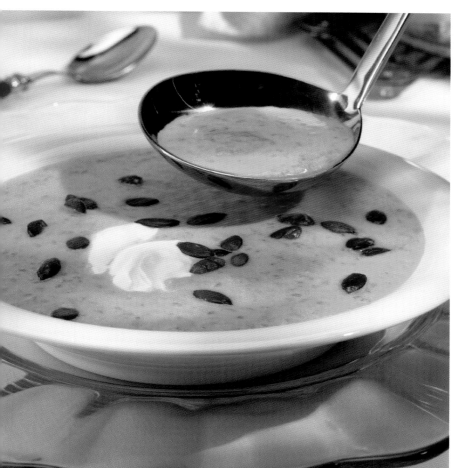

NUTRIENTS PER SERVING

Calories: 200

Total Fat: 8g	
Saturated Fat: 1g	
Cholesterol: 30mg	
Sodium: 350mg	
Total Carbohydrate: 28g	
Dietary Fiber: 10g	
Sugars: 11g	
Protein: 7g	

% Daily Value
Vit A: 260%   Vit C: 70%
Calcium: 10%   Iron: 20%

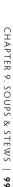

Jamaican Red Pea Soup

A Jamaican classic, which my husband loves! I keep the bones in the chicken legs for him, as he says "soup bone sweet." Cut the fat by removing the skin. This soup traditionally calls for white flour dumplings, but I have taken them out. Feel free to serve this over brown rice.

INGREDIENTS

- 4 bone-in, skinless chicken legs
- 3 cups dry kidney beans
- 1 large sweet potato, peeled and cubed
- 2 white onions, chopped
- 2 scallions, chopped
- 2 carrots, chopped
- 1 hot pepper, preferably scotch bonnet, seeded and chopped
- 2 tsp dried thyme
- 1 tsp freshly ground black pepper
- 4 cups low sodium chicken broth
- 1 can (14 oz) light (or lite) coconut milk

JNL'S FUN, FIT FOODIE TIP: Use gloves to take the seeds out of the pepper, as that's where most of the heat is. Don't touch your eyes, and wash your hands promptly after touching the pepper.

DIRECTIONS

1. Place the chicken, beans, sweet potato, onion, scallion, carrots, hot pepper, thyme, black pepper into a pressure cooker. Pour in the broth and coconut milk.

2. Set the pressure cooker for 20 minutes. Check the beans, if still firm, set to cook for another 10 minutes. Shred the chicken from the legs (discard the bones) and stir into the soup. Serves 8.

NUTRIENTS PER SERVING

Calories: 420

Total Fat: 8g	
Saturated Fat: 4g	
Cholesterol: 45mg	
Sodium: 220mg	
Total Carbohydrate: 54g	
Dietary Fiber: 12g	
Sugars: 6g	
Protein: 31g	

% Daily Value
Vit A: 4%   Vit C: 35%
Calcium: 10%   Iron: 35%
Excellent source of thiamin, niacin, vitamin B6, folate, magnesium, selenium and zinc.

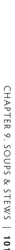

Thai Coconut Shrimp Soup

Bold and flavorful, this soup is a terrific option to have on hand if friends stop by.

INGREDIENTS:

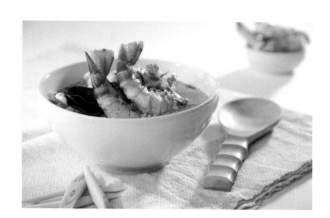

- 1 lb medium raw shrimp, peeled and de-veined
- 1 lb shiitake mushrooms, sliced
- 2 cans (14 oz each) light (or Lite) coconut milk
- 2 cups water
- ¼ cup lime juice
- ¼ cup brown sugar substitute (or honey to taste)
- 3 tbsp fish sauce
- 1 1-inch piece ginger, thinly sliced
- 1 ½ tsp lemongrass paste
- 1 tsp Thai curry paste or curry powder
- 1 tsp dried red pepper flakes
- Thinly sliced scallion

DIRECTIONS:

1. Stir shrimp, mushrooms, coconut milk, water, lime juice, sugar substitute, fish sauce, ginger, lemongrass paste, curry paste and red pepper flakes together in a pressure cooker.

2. Set pressure cooker to cook for 10 minutes. Garnish each bowl of soup with scallion. Serves 6.

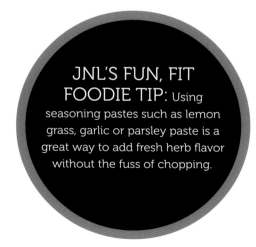

JNL'S FUN, FIT FOODIE TIP: Using seasoning pastes such as lemon grass, garlic or parsley paste is a great way to add fresh herb flavor without the fuss of chopping.

NUTRIENTS PER SERVING

Calories: 190

Total Fat: 7g	
Saturated Fat: 6g	
Cholesterol: 80mg	
Sodium: 770mg	
Total Carbohydrate: 21g	
Dietary Fiber: 1g	
Sugars: 10g	
Protein: 11g	

% Daily Value
Vit A: 0%   Vit C: 8%
Calcium: 2%   Iron: 10%
Excellent source of selenium.

Homemade & Heart Healthy Fresh Vegetable Soup

Nothing warms your heart (and belly) like a nice, big bowl of fresh vegetable soup. I pick my vegetables from my local farmers market, and get organic whenever I can. By not overcooking the fresh vegetables, you can maintain most of the vegetables' nutrients. This is a vegetarian soup, but you can create Vegetable Beef soup simply by adding ground beef to the pressure cooker.

INGREDIENTS:

- 4 cups low sodium vegetable broth
- ½ cup diced carrots
- ½ cup chopped green beans
- ½ cup fresh corn kernels off the cob
- ½ cup diced celery
- ½ cup small broccoli florets
- 2 Roma tomatoes, diced
- 1 sprig fresh thyme
- JAT freshly ground black pepper

DIRECTIONS:

1. Combine vegetable broth, carrots, green beans, corn, celery, broccoli, tomatoes, thyme and pepper in a pressure cooker. Set pressure cooker to cook for 10 minutes. Discard the sprig of thyme before serving. Serves 2.

NUTRIENTS PER SERVING

Calories: 100

Total Fat: 0.5g	
Saturated Fat: 0g	
Cholesterol: 0mg	
Sodium: 240mg	
Total Carbohydrate: 24g	
Dietary Fiber: 4g	
Sugars: 10g	
Protein: 4g	

% Daily Value
Vit A: 15%   Vit C: 60%
Calcium: 6%   Iron: 8%

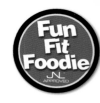

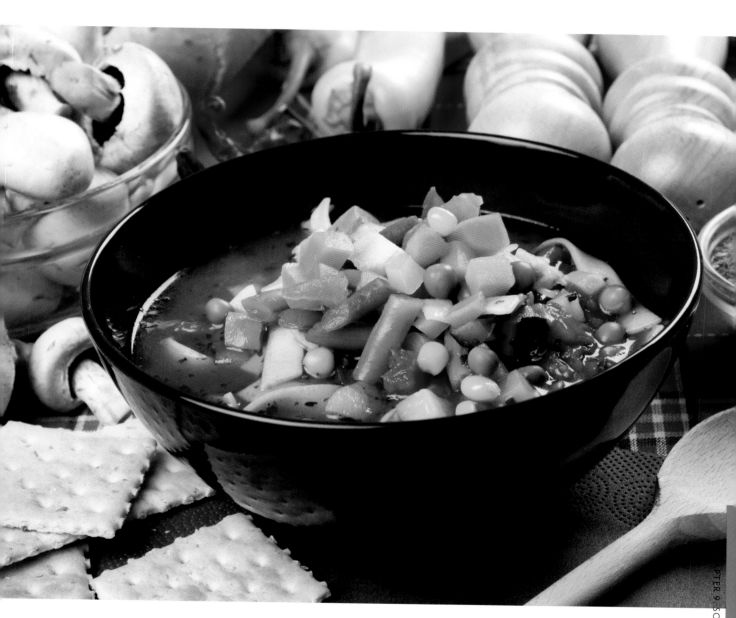

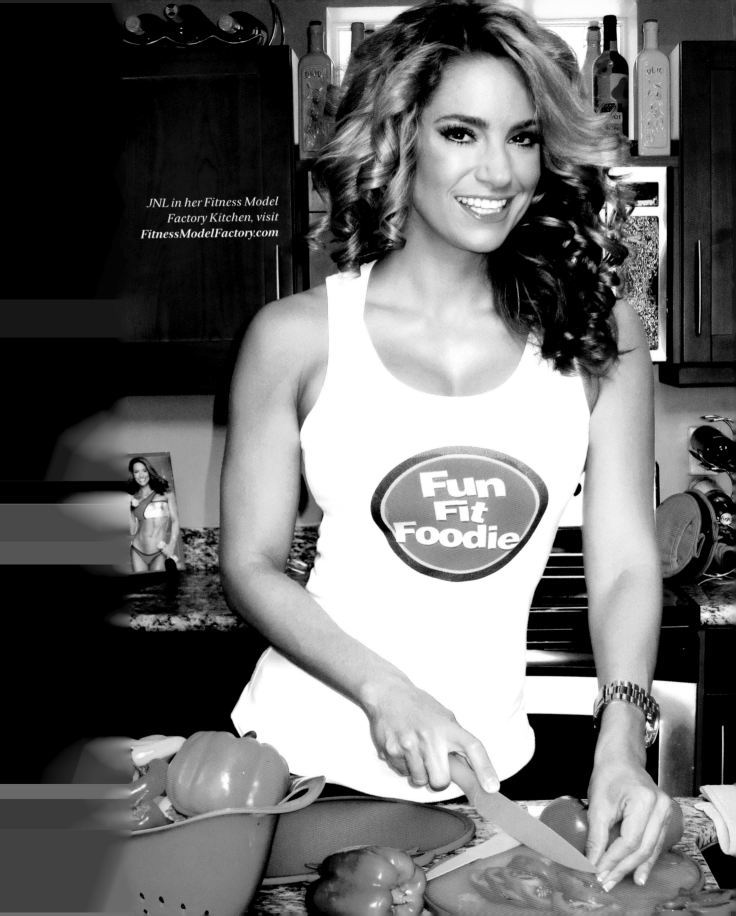

Fun
Fit
Foodie

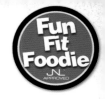

Strawberry and Blueberry Spinach Salad

A super-easy, refreshing summer salad loaded with antioxidant-rich foods. If I don't have light salad dressings on hand, I simply whisk a little water into regular salad dressing to make it go farther.

INGREDIENTS:

- 1 bag (6 oz) baby spinach leaves
- 4 cups sliced fresh strawberries
- 1 cup fresh blueberries
- 3 tbsp light poppy-seed style salad dressing

DIRECTIONS:

1. In a large bowl, toss the spinach with the strawberries and blueberries; pour over the poppy seed dressing onto the spinach mixture and toss to coat. Serves 4.

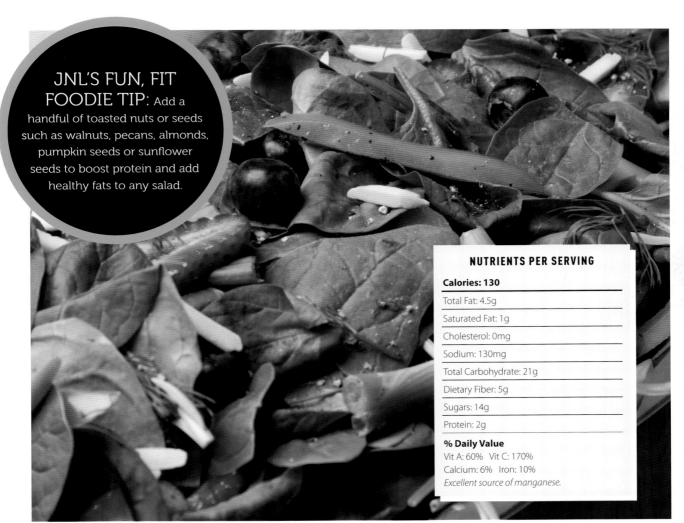

JNL'S FUN, FIT FOODIE TIP: Add a handful of toasted nuts or seeds such as walnuts, pecans, almonds, pumpkin seeds or sunflower seeds to boost protein and add healthy fats to any salad.

NUTRIENTS PER SERVING

Calories: 130

Total Fat: 4.5g	
Saturated Fat: 1g	
Cholesterol: 0mg	
Sodium: 130mg	
Total Carbohydrate: 21g	
Dietary Fiber: 5g	
Sugars: 14g	
Protein: 2g	

% Daily Value
Vit A: 60% Vit C: 170%
Calcium: 6% Iron: 10%
Excellent source of manganese.

Caribbean Shrimp, Papaya & Avocado Salad

This salad was introduced to me, when I first moved to the beautiful, magical city of Miami. Being Italian, I love the Mediterranean flavor of the fresh shrimp salad, combined with avocado. This is a Cuban staple and I am honored to share it with my fellow Fun, Fit Foodies!

INGREDIENTS:

- ¾ cup extra-virgin olive oil
- ¼ cup fresh lemon juice
- ¼ tsp freshly ground black pepper (approx.)
- ¼ tsp ground cumin
- 1 tbsp finely chopped fresh parsley
- JAT sea salt
- 1 lb medium shrimp, peeled and de-veined
- 1 large ripe papaya, peeled, seeded and thinly sliced
- 1 large, ripe avocado, peeled, pitted and thinly sliced
- ½ small red onion, finely chopped

DIRECTIONS:

1. Whisk the olive oil, lemon juice, parsley, pepper, cumin and salt (to taste) in a small bowl. Store tightly covered in the fridge for up to 4 days.

2. Bring a saucepan of salted water to a boil. Add the shrimp; simmer for 3 minutes or until shrimp are pink. Drain and rinse the shrimp under cold running water until completely cooled. Drain well.

3. Place an equal portion of shrimp in the center of 6 individual bowls; arrange the avocado and papaya along the sides. Sprinkle with the onion and additional pepper (to taste). Drizzle each portion with 2 to 3 tsp of the dressing. (Reserve remaining dressing for another purpose). Serves 6.

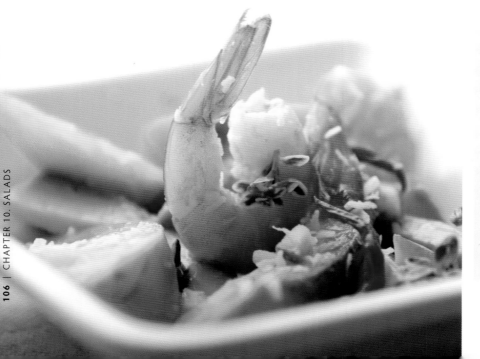

NUTRIENTS PER SERVING

Calories: 180

Total Fat: 12g	
Saturated Fat: 2g	
Cholesterol: 80mg	
Sodium: 110mg	
Total Carbohydrate: 11g	
Dietary Fiber: 4g	
Sugars: 5g	
Protein: 10g	

% Daily Value
Vit A: 0%   Vit C: 80%
Calcium: 4%   Iron: 8%
Excellent source of selenium.

Barley Vegetable Salad with Feta

Barley is usually used in soups or stews, but I like to use it to "beef" up a delicious vegetable salad sprinkled with feta. Dig in!

INGREDIENTS:

- 1 ½ cups chopped carrots
- 1 green bell pepper, seeded and diced
- 1 cup cooked pearl barley
- 1 cup shredded red cabbage
- ½ cup minced red onion
- ¼ cup minced sun-dried tomatoes
- 1 tbsp red wine vinegar
- 2 tsp horseradish mustard
- 1 tsp extra virgin olive oil
- JAT freshly ground black pepper
- JAT cayenne pepper
- 2 tbsp crumbled feta cheese

DIRECTIONS:

1. Toss the carrots with the green pepper, barley, cabbage, onion and sun-dried tomatoes.

2. Whisk vinegar with mustard, oil, black and cayenne peppers until combined. Pour over the vegetable barley mixture and stir to coat. Garnish with feta cheese. Serves 4.

JNL'S FUN, FIT FOODIE TIP:

Hands down, barley is one of the best whole grains for you. It has more fiber than brown rice. One cup of whole-grain barley flour has nearly 15 grams of dietary fiber, and just two grams of fat. But it isn't just the volume of fiber; it is the type of fiber that is important. Barley has a very high level of viscous soluble fiber (called Beta-glucan). Studies have shown that a diet high in viscous fiber such as Beta-glucan helps to lower blood LDL cholesterol (so-called "bad" cholesterol) levels, a risk factor for heart disease. Such diets may also help stabilize blood glucose levels, which could benefit people with non-insulin dependent diabetes. Whole-grain barley also contains high levels of minerals and important vitamins including calcium, magnesium, phosphorus, potassium, vitamin A, vitamin E, niacin and folate. The vitamin E found in whole-grain barley contains both tocopherols and tocotrienols, powerful antioxidants that, research indicates, may reduce the risk of certain cancers and help lower blood pressure.

NUTRIENTS PER SERVING

Calories: 130
Total Fat: 2.5g
Saturated Fat: 1g
Cholesterol: 4mg
Sodium: 210mg
Total Carbohydrate: 23g
Dietary Fiber: 4g
Sugars: 6g
Protein: 3g

% Daily Value
Vit A: 20%   Vit C: 90%
Calcium: 8%   Iron: 6%

Pear & Pecan Chicken Salad

The most amazing blend of sweet apples and pears, tender grilled lean chicken breast, juicy grapes adorned with real chunks of blue cheese and toasted pecans...yum!

INGREDIENTS:

- 1 cup apple juice
- 2 tbsp cider vinegar
- 1 tsp extra-virgin olive oil
- ¼ tsp freshly ground black pepper
- 10 cups mixed gourmet salad greens (about 10 oz)
- 12 oz sliced, pre-grilled chicken breast
- 1 cup seedless red grapes, halved
- 1 medium McIntosh apple, cored and cut into 18 wedges
- 1 medium Bartlett pear, cored and cut into 18 wedges
- 3 tbsp chopped, toasted pecans
- 2 tbsp crumbled blue cheese

DIRECTIONS:

1. Place apple juice in a small saucepan set over medium-high heat; bring to a boil. Cook, for 10 minutes or until the juice is reduced to about 3 tbsp. Whisk the reduced apple juice with the vinegar, oil, and pepper until combined.

2. Toss the mixed greens with the chicken, grapes, apple and pear in a large salad bowl. Drizzle with the apple dressing mixture; toss gently to coat. Sprinkle nuts and blue cheese on top. Serves 4.

NUTRIENTS PER SERVING

Calories: 200

Total Fat: 6g
Saturated Fat: 1g
Cholesterol: 35mg
Sodium: 290mg
Total Carbohydrate: 25g
Dietary Fiber: 3g
Sugars: 18g
Protein: 16g

% Daily Value
Vit A: 20%   Vit C: 35%
Calcium: 8% Iron: 4%

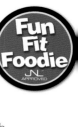

Cucumber, Tomato and Feta Salad

Another fresh and cool salad to serve along-side grilled lean chicken breast, steak or fish. If you use English cucumber you skip the peeling and seeding step and get an additional boost of fiber.

INGREDIENTS:

- 2 tomatoes, sliced
- 1 ½ cucumbers, peeled, seeded and sliced
- JAT freshly ground black pepper
- 2 tbsp red wine vinegar
- 2 tbsp olive oil
- ⅓ cup crumbled feta cheese

DIRECTIONS:

1. Combine tomatoes and cucumber in a large bowl. Season with pepper. Add vinegar and olive oil. Toss to coat. Arrange on a platter and sprinkle evenly with feta. Serves 4.

JNL'S FUN, FIT FOODIE TIP: Eating water-based foods such as cucumber, lettuce, grapes and watermelon is a great way to supplement your water intake throughout the day.

NUTRIENTS PER SERVING

Calories: 120

Total Fat: 10g	
Saturated Fat: 3g	
Cholesterol: 10mg	
Sodium: 150mg	
Total Carbohydrate: 6g	
Dietary Fiber: 2g	
Sugars: 4g	
Protein: 3g	

% Daily Value
Vit A: 4%   Vit C: 25%
Calcium: 8%   Iron: 4%

Apple & Walnut Endive Salad with Fresh Cranberry Dressing

Using concentrated juice in your salad dressings is a great way to add bold flavor without extra fat. This elegant, colorful salad is a terrific accompaniment to roasted turkey.

INGREDIENTS:

- 2 tbsp extra-virgin olive oil
- 2 tbsp thawed, frozen cranberry juice concentrate
- 1 tbsp white wine vinegar
- JAT freshly ground black pepper
- 3 heads Belgian endive, thinly sliced
- 2 apples, cored and chopped (peel on)
- ½ cup chopped fresh cranberries
- ¼ cup coarsely chopped, toasted walnuts

DIRECTIONS:

1. Whisk the oil with the cranberry juice concentrate and vinegar until well combined. Season with pepper.

2. Toss the endive and apples in medium bowl. Pour the dressing over and toss to coat. Sprinkle with cranberries and walnuts. Serves 4.

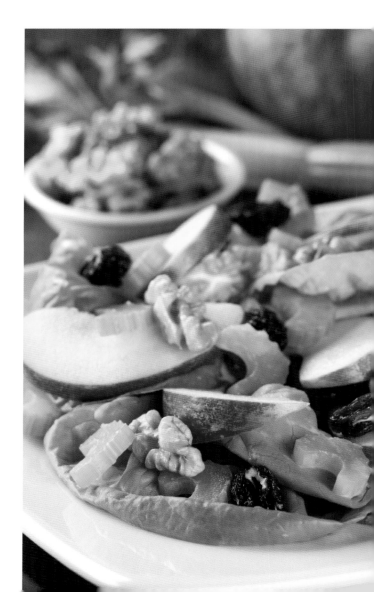

NUTRIENTS PER SERVING

Calories: 170

Total Fat: 12g	
Saturated Fat: 1.5g	
Cholesterol: 0mg	
Sodium: 0mg	
Total Carbohydrate: 18g	
Dietary Fiber: 4g	
Sugars: 12g	
Protein: 2g	

% Daily Value
Vit A: 0%   Vit C: 15%
Calcium: 2%   Iron: 2%

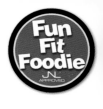

Blackened Shrimp with Corn and Black Bean Salad

A fiesta of colorful ingredients tossed with a zesty dressing. You can also use the corn and black bean salad as a side for grilled steak or chicken.

INGREDIENTS:

- ¼ cup balsamic vinegar
- 2 tbsp extra-virgin olive oil
- ½ tsp freshly ground black pepper
- ½ tsp ground cumin
- ½ tsp chili powder
- 5 dashes hot sauce
- 1 can (15 oz) black beans, rinsed and drained
- 1 can (8.75 oz) sweet corn, rinsed and drained
- 1 small red bell pepper, seeded and chopped
- ½ red onion, chopped
- 1 lb medium shrimp, peeled and de-veined
- JAT Mrs. Dash Extra Spicy salt-free seasoning
- 3 tbsp chopped fresh cilantro
- Lime wedges

DIRECTIONS:

1. Whisk the balsamic vinegar with the oil, black pepper, cumin, chili powder and hot sauce until combined. Add the black beans, corn, red pepper and red onion; toss to coat. Chill for 15 minutes to meld the flavors.

2. Meanwhile, lightly coat a medium skillet with nonstick cooking spray; set over medium-high heat. Add the shrimp and stir-fry until pink. Sprinkle with salt-free seasoning to taste. Divide the black bean salad between 4 serving plates. Top each with an equal portion of warm shrimp. Garnish with cilantro and lime wedges. Serves 4.

NUTRIENTS PER SERVING

Calories: 280	
Total Fat: 9g	
Saturated Fat: 1g	
Cholesterol: 120mg	
Sodium: 630mg	
Total Carbohydrate: 29g	
Dietary Fiber: 6g	
Sugars: 7g	
Protein: 19g	

% Daily Value
Vit A: 5%   Vit C: 70%
Calcium: 6%   Iron: 20%
Excellent source of selenium.

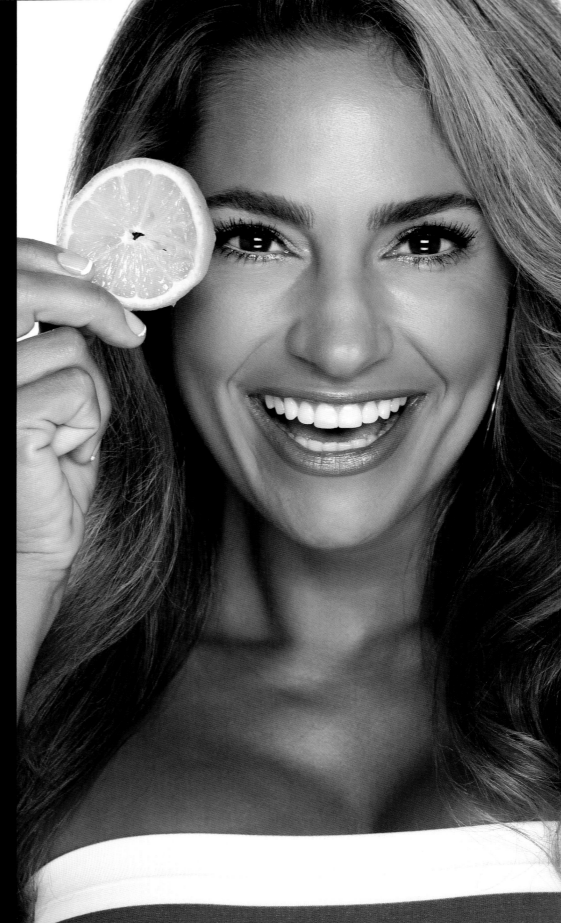

11. SIDES, STARTERS, & HEALTHY SNACKS

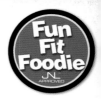

Grandpa Rudy's Stuffed Artichokes

My dad, Rudolpho Siciliano, Rudy for short, was the first one ever to introduce me to the amazing artichoke. Funny as it sounds, I can remember distinctly this being the very first vegetable that I had ever seen. As a baby, I can recall all of my Italian family in the kitchen together, stuffing artichokes, then steaming them, and then peeling one leaf off at a time, to get to the "heart" of the artichoke. Now being a mom myself, and a devout Fun, Fit Foodie, I am thrilled to know just how healthy they are!

INGREDIENTS:

- 2 cups whole wheat breadcrumbs
- ¼ cup olive oil
- JAT freshly ground black pepper
- JAT Mrs. Dash Italian Seasoning
- 4 whole artichokes, trimmed
- 1 cup white wine
- ½ cup low sodium vegetable or chicken broth

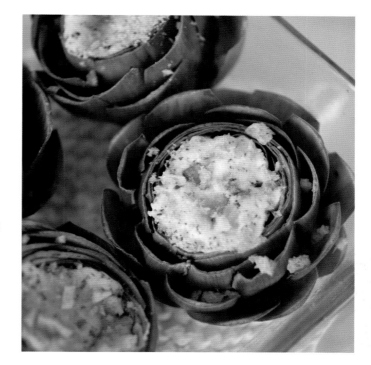

DIRECTIONS:

1. Toss the breadcrumbs with the olive oil, pepper and Italian seasoning to combine. Stuff an equal portion of this mixture into the centre of each artichoke.

2. Pour the wine and broth into a pressure cooker. Arrange artichokes, stem-side-up, into the pressure cooker. Set the pressure cooker for 15 minutes. Transfer the artichokes to a serving platter. Drizzle the stuffing with some of the hot cooking liquid to moisten. Serves 4.

JNL'S FUN, FIT FOODIE TIP: Artichokes are an excellent source of dietary fiber, magnesium, and the trace mineral chromium. They are a very good source of vitamin C, folic acid, biotin, and the trace mineral manganese. They also contain the nutrients niacin, riboflavin, thiamine, vitamin A and potassium.

NUTRIENTS PER SERVING
(1 artichoke)

Calories: 310

Total Fat: 16g	
Saturated Fat: 2g	
Cholesterol: 0mg	
Sodium: 320mg	
Total Carbohydrate: 36g	
Dietary Fiber: 8g	
Sugars: 5g	
Protein: 9g	

% Daily Value
Vit A: 0%   Vit C: 20%
Calcium: 8%   Iron: 15%

Sweet Potato Casserole

I was raised in the Deep South, and brought up being fed a mix of fusion foods; from those that stemmed from my Italian heritage to Southern staples like sweet potato casserole. I gained a love for the sweetness of this dish, but I also gained a pound or two when I ate it! So I gave it my Fun, Fit Foodie makeover. By leaving out the traditional stick of butter and marshmallows, and adding the heart-healthy pecans on top, I gave it a complete, healthy remix.

INGREDIENTS:

- 3 medium sweet potatoes
- 3 egg whites
- ½ cup skim milk
- 1 tbsp sunflower oil
- 1 tbsp honey
- 2 tsp finely grated orange zest
- 1 tsp vanilla extract

Topping:

- ½ cup whole-wheat flour
- ½ cup chopped pecans
- ⅓ cup packed brown sugar substitute
- 2 tbsp applesauce
- 1 tbsp sunflower oil
- 4 tsp thawed, frozen orange juice concentrate

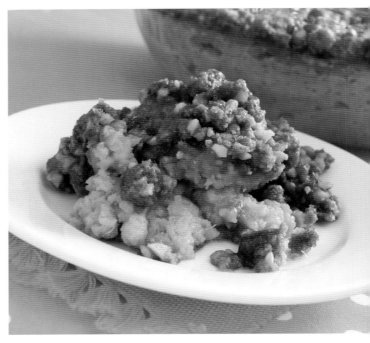

DIRECTIONS

1. Preheat the oven to 400°F. Bake the sweet potatoes for about 45 minutes or until tender. Cool until easy to handle; peel and mash the sweet potatoes. Meanwhile, lightly coat a baking dish with nonstick cooking spray.

2. Whisk the egg whites with the milk, oil, honey, orange zest and vanilla in a medium bowl. Fold in the mashed sweet potato until well combined. Spread the sweet potato mixture into the prepared baking dish.

3. Topping: Combine the flour, pecans and sugar substitute in a bowl. Blend in the applesauce, oil and orange juice concentrate using a fork or your fingertips until crumbly. Sprinkle evenly over the sweet potato mixture. Bake the casserole for 35 to 45 minutes or until completely until heated through and topping is lightly browned. Serves 6.

NUTRIENTS PER SERVING

Calories: 270

Total Fat: 11g	
Saturated Fat: 1g	
Cholesterol: 0mg	
Sodium: 45mg	
Total Carbohydrate: 37g	
Dietary Fiber: 4g	
Sugars: 21g	
Protein: 5g	

% Daily Value
Vit A: 35%   Vit C: 30%
Calcium: 4%   Iron: 6%
Excellent source of manganese.

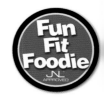

"No Stirring" Risotto

Easy-to-make risotto? Yes, right here — and you are not dreaming! Surprise your family and friends with this gourmet meal made simple. Serve as a side dish at lunch with your grilled fish or chicken meals.

INGREDIENTS:

- 2 tbsp olive oil
- 6 oz mixed wild mushrooms (such as cremini, oyster, shitake and/or porcini)
- ⅓ cup chopped onion
- 1 tbsp minced garlic
- 1 cup Arborio rice
- 1 ½ cups water
- ½ cup dry white wine
- JAT fresh or dried thyme
- ¼ cup chopped fresh parsley
- ¾ cup shredded Romano cheese, divided
- ¼ cup 2% milk

DIRECTIONS:

1. Heat the oil in saucepan set over medium heat. Add the mushrooms, onion and garlic. Cook, stirring, for 5 minutes or until tender.

2. Stir in the rice until well-combined. Pour in the water and wine. Bring to boil; cover. Reduce the heat to low. Simmer for 20 minutes or until the rice is tender. Stir in the thyme and parsley. Stir in ½ cup of the cheese and the milk. Serve with remaining cheese on the side. Serves 6.

NUTRIENTS PER SERVING

Calories: 230	
Total Fat: 8g	
Saturated Fat: 3g	
Cholesterol: 15mg	
Sodium: 160mg	
Total Carbohydrate: 29g	
Dietary Fiber: 1g	
Sugars: 2g	
Protein: 7g	

% Daily Value
Vit A: 2%   Vit C: 8%
Calcium: 15%   Iron: 4%

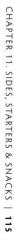

Steamed Asparagus with Lemon

Asparagus is an amazing, healthy detox vegetable that gets rid of extra water weight. It's the perfect Fun, Fit Foodie side dish. Not only is it easy to make, it has few ingredients. Completely foolproof!

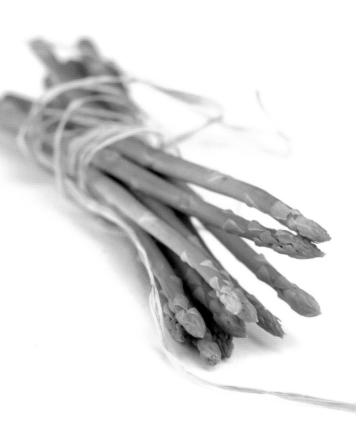

INGREDIENTS:

- 2 lb fresh asparagus, trimmed
- 2 tbsp extra virgin olive oil
- 2 tsp fresh lemon juice
- JAT sea salt and freshly ground pepper

DIRECTIONS:

1. Steam asparagus in steamer basket set over boiling water for 10 to 15 minutes or until asparagus are tender-crisp. (Do not overcook.) Remove from the steamer basket; allow to cool for 2 minutes. Wrap asparagus in paper towel and blot to remove excess water. Transfer to a serving dish.

2. Drizzle olive oil and lemon juice over asparagus. Sprinkle with salt and pepper. Serve immediately. Serves 6.

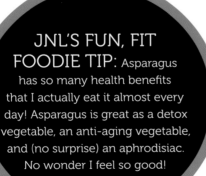

JNL'S FUN, FIT FOODIE TIP: Asparagus has so many health benefits that I actually eat it almost every day! Asparagus is great as a detox vegetable, an anti-aging vegetable, and (no surprise) an aphrodisiac. No wonder I feel so good!

NUTRIENTS PER SERVING

Calories: 70

Total Fat: 4.5g	
Saturated Fat: 0.5g	
Cholesterol: 0mg	
Sodium: 100mg	
Total Carbohydrate: 6g	
Dietary Fiber: 3g	
Sugars: 3g	
Protein: 3g	

% Daily Value
Vit A: 4%   Vit C: 15%
Calcium: 4%   Iron: 20%

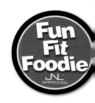

Roasted Red Peppers in Olive Oil and Garlic with Grilled Shrimp

These peppers are powerhouses packed with an incredible amount of vitamin C, giving you over 300% of your RDA per serving! Shrimp is a low-fat, low-calorie protein source, which is high in selenium (a nutrient needed in small doses for overall health). And certainly everyone knows the healthful benefits of olive oil and garlic! So, start your meal off right with this appetizer.

INGREDIENTS:

- 4 large red bell peppers, halved and seeded
- 1 tbsp olive oil, divided
- 2 tsp balsamic vinegar
- JAT salt-free Italian seasoning
- 24 medium fresh shrimp, peeled and de-veined
- 1 clove garlic, minced
- 2 tbsp finely chopped fresh basil
- Toasted whole grain baguette

DIRECTIONS:

1. Preheat the broiler to high. Rub the peppers with 1 tsp of the olive oil and place on a cookie sheet. Broil the peppers, turning as needed, for 3 to 5 minutes, or until skin is charred and bubbly.

2. Transfer the peppers to a plastic bag (this trick will allow steam to loosen the skins making them easier to peel). Once cool enough to handle, rub off the skin and discard along with the seeds. Chop the peppers and toss with balsamic vinegar and Italian seasoning.

3. Heat the remaining olive oil in a large skillet. Add the garlic and shrimp and cook, stirring for 3 to 4 minutes or until shrimp are pink. Pile the shrimp on a platter, arrange the peppers on the side. Sprinkle all over with basil. Serve with toasted baguette. Serves 6.

NUTRIENTS PER SERVING

Calories: 170

Total Fat: 4g	
Saturated Fat: 0.5g	
Cholesterol: 85mg	
Sodium: 240mg	
Total Carbohydrate: 21g	
Dietary Fiber: 6g	
Sugars: 8g	
Protein: 14g	

% Daily Value
Vit A: 15% Vit C: 350%
Calcium: 20% Iron: 15%
Excellent source of selenium.

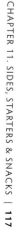

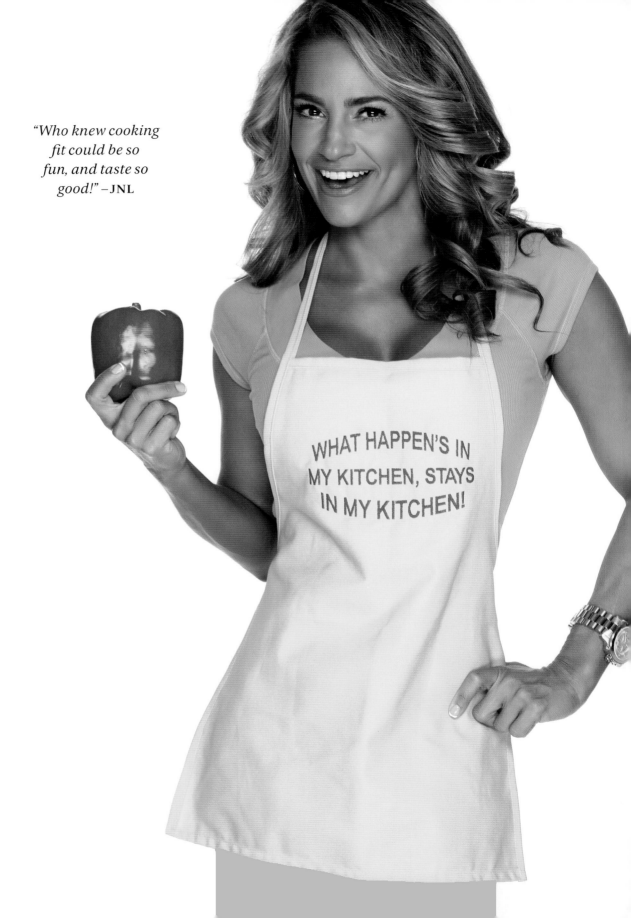

"Who knew cooking fit could be so fun, and taste so good!" –JNL

WHAT HAPPEN'S IN MY KITCHEN, STAYS IN MY KITCHEN!

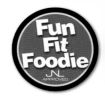

Siciliano Steamed Mussels in a White Wine Broth

When I was growing up, on Sundays my dad would cook all day long. He would often serve this family favorite as one of the appetizers. This recipe includes a little butter, salt and cream, but as an appetizer, a little goes a long way.

INGREDIENTS:

- 1 tbsp olive oil
- 1 tbsp butter
- ½ cup sliced shallots
- JAT sea salt and fresh ground pepper
- 2 cloves garlic, minced
- 1 cup low sodium chicken broth
- ½ cup white wine
- 1 ½ lb mussels, cleaned and trimmed of beards
- 1 tbsp heavy cream
- 2 tbsp chopped fresh parsley
- Lemon wedges
- Crusty whole grain bread

JNL'S FUN, FIT FOODIE TIP: Mussels are high in B12 vitamins and provide a readily absorbed source of many other B & C vitamins, amino acids, vital minerals including iron, manganese, phosphorus, potassium, selenium and zinc. They have more omega 3 fatty acids than any other shellfish and far more than any other popular meat choice today. Mussels are also low in sodium, fat and cholesterol but high in protein. Fifteen mussels provide the equivalent protein of a 6 oz steak.

DIRECTIONS:

1. Heat the oil and butter in a large pot set over medium heat. Add shallots and season with salt and pepper; sauté for 5 minutes. Add the garlic and cook for 1 minute.

2. Pour in the wine and chicken broth. Add the mussels. Cover and steam the mussels for about 10 minutes or until all the mussels are open. (Discard any that do not open.)

3. Use a slotted spoon to transfer the mussels to a serving bowl. Stir the cream and parsley into the cooking liquid; spoon over the mussels. Serve with lemon wedges and crusty bread on the side. Serves 4.

NUTRIENTS PER SERVING
(mussels and broth only)

Calories: 200

Total Fat: 10g	
Saturated Fat: 3.5g	
Cholesterol: 45mg	
Sodium: 430mg	
Total Carbohydrate: 8g	
Dietary Fiber: 0g	
Sugars: 1g	
Protein: 15g	

% Daily Value
Vit A: 4% Vit C: 20%
Calcium: 4% Iron: 25%
Excellent source of vitamin B12 and selenium.

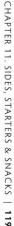

Teriyaki Salmon Sliders with Spicy Broccoli Slaw

These sliders are a HIT, even with folks who don't care for fish. The bite-sized buns and the barbecue sauce put a new, fresh spin on salmon, which is too often snubbed as a "diet food." These fun and easy-to-whip-up sliders will have your entire family or party guests raving!

INGREDIENTS:

- 4 small boneless salmon steak, cut into two equal portions
- ¼ cup Asian-style barbecue sauce
- 12 whole-grain mini sandwich rolls
- 12 oz Asian broccoli slaw salad mix (such as Eat Smart® Asian Salad Kit)

DIRECTIONS:

1. Brush the barbecue sauce over the salmon. Marinate for at least 2 hours. Preheat an indoor or outdoor grill to medium. Add the salmon and cook, to your preferred doneness.

2. Meanwhile, toss the salad kit according to package directions. Place the salmon on the slider buns and garnish with the slaw. Makes 12 sliders.

JNL'S FUN, FIT FOODIE TIP: I love the Eat Smart Salad Kits! This one contains shredded green cabbage, broccoli, carrots and red cabbage, as well as chow mein noodles, sliced almonds and a sesame dressing. Simply open, mix and enjoy! How simple is that? Less time in the kitchen, and more time with your friends and family, enjoying the meal together.

NUTRIENTS PER SERVING
(2 sliders)

Calories: 460	
Total Fat: 19g	
Saturated Fat: 2.5g	
Cholesterol: 55mg	
Sodium: 590mg	
Total Carbohydrate: 44g	
Dietary Fiber: 4g	
Sugars: 13g	
Protein: 30g	

% Daily Value
Vit A: 8%   Vit C: 35%
Calcium: 10%   Iron: 15%
Excellent source of niacin, vitamin B12 and vitamin D.

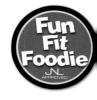

HOLY MOLY Guacamole

A wholesome, multipurpose condiment that you can serve with whole grain tortilla chips, or as a compliment to any dish you wish! Ideal for the "Latina Loca" Beef Bowl Salad *(on page 74)*.

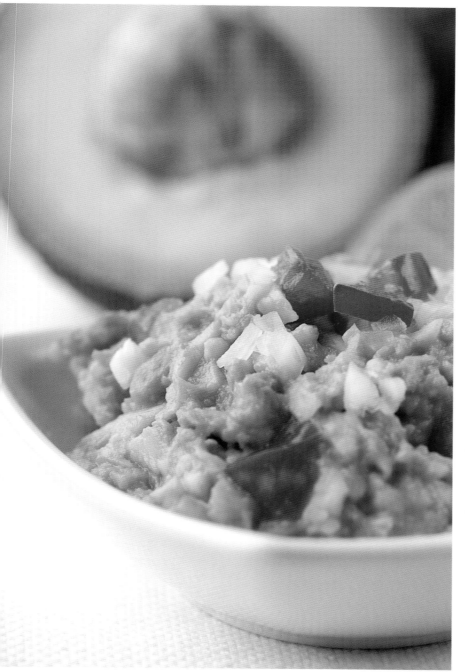

INGREDIENTS:

- 3 large avocados, halved and pitted
- 1 lime, juiced
- 2 Roma tomatoes, diced
- 1 tbsp finely chopped cilantro
- 1 tsp garlic purée
- JAT freshly ground black pepper

DIRECTIONS:

1. Mash the avocado with the lime juice in a large bowl (I like to leave it a tad chunky for extra texture). Fold in the tomatoes, cilantro and garlic until combined. Season with pepper (to taste). Makes about 3 cups.

NUTRIENTS PER SERVING
(2 tbsp)

Calories: 41	
Total Fat: 4g	
Saturated Fat: 0.5g	
Cholesterol: 0mg	
Sodium: 5mg	
Total Carbohydrate: 2g	
Dietary Fiber: 2g	
Sugars: 0g	
Protein: 1g	

% Daily Value
Vit A: 0%   Vit C: 6%
Calcium: 0%   Iron: 0%

Blueberry Banana Vanilla Shake

A protein shake is a terrific pick-me-up before a workout or as a meal replacement when you are on the run. Raspberries or strawberries can be used instead of the blueberries.

INGREDIENTS:

- 1 cup skim milk
- 1 cup ice cubes (approx.)
- ½ banana
- ¼ cup fresh or frozen blueberries
- 1 scoop vanilla protein shake mix

DIRECTIONS:

1. Combine milk, ice, banana, blueberries and shake mix in a blender. Blend until smooth. (Adjust consistency with extra ice or water as preferred). Serves 1 as a meal replacement, 2 as a snack.

JNL'S FUN, FIT FOODIE TIP:

You can replace some of the ice if you use frozen sliced bananas instead.

NUTRIENTS PER SERVING
(1 shake)

Calories: 300

Total Fat: 4g	
Saturated Fat: 1.5g	
Cholesterol: 55mg	
Sodium: 220mg	
Total Carbohydrate: 37g	
Dietary Fiber: 3g	
Sugars: 24g	
Protein: 30g	

% Daily Value
Vit A: 10%   Vit C: 15%
Calcium: 45%   Iron: 4%
Excellent source of riboflavin, vitamin B12, vitamin D.

Fruit Smoothie with Coconut Oil

Start the day off with a breakfast bang! Wash down your vitamins with a rich, delicious protein smoothie with coconut oil. The strawberries can be replaced with any fruit you have in the fridge at the time.

INGREDIENTS:

- 1 cup skim milk
- ½ cup fresh or frozen strawberries
- 2 tbsp room temperature virgin coconut oil
- 1 scoop vanilla protein shake mix
- 3 ice cubes

DIRECTIONS:

1. Combine milk, strawberries, coconut oil, shake mix and ice cubes in a blender. Blend until smooth. (Adjust consistency with extra ice or water as preferred.) Serves 1 as a meal replacement, 2 as a snack.

NUTRIENTS PER SERVING
(1 shake)

Calories: 250

Total Fat: 16g	
Saturated Fat: 13g	
Cholesterol: 25mg	
Sodium: 110mg	
Total Carbohydrate: 13g	
Dietary Fiber: 1g	
Sugars: 9g	
Protein: 15g	

% Daily Value
Vit A: 5%   Vit C: 35%
Calcium: 25%   Iron: 2%

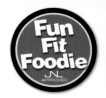

Iced Chai Protein Shake

The coffee-house flavor of Chai that you love, but in a satisfying nutrition shake.

INGREDIENTS:

- 1 cup water
- ½ cup Chai tea concentrate
- ¼ cup orange juice
- ¼ cup cranberry juice
- 1 scoop Vanilla or Chai tea flavored protein shake mix
- JAT ground cinnamon
- JAT ground ginger

DIRECTIONS:

1. Combine water, Chai concentrate, orange juice, cranberry juice, shake mix, cinnamon and ginger in a blender. Blend until smooth. Serves 1 as a meal replacement, 2 as a snack.

JNL'S FUN, FIT FOODIE TIP: The main differences between virgin coconut oil and refined coconut oil are the scent and taste. All virgin coconut oils retain the fresh scent and taste of coconuts, while the refined coconut oils have a bland taste due to the refining process.

JNL'S FUN, FIT FOODIE TIP: You can usually find Chai tea concentrate in the coffee and tea section of your grocery store.

NUTRIENTS PER SERVING
(1 shake)

Calories: 290

Total Fat: 3.5g
Saturated Fat: 1g
Cholesterol: 50mg
Sodium: 140mg
Total Carbohydrate: 41g
Dietary Fiber: 1g
Sugars: 33g
Protein: 21g

% Daily Value
Vit A: 0%   Vit C: 50%
Calcium: 15%   Iron: 2%

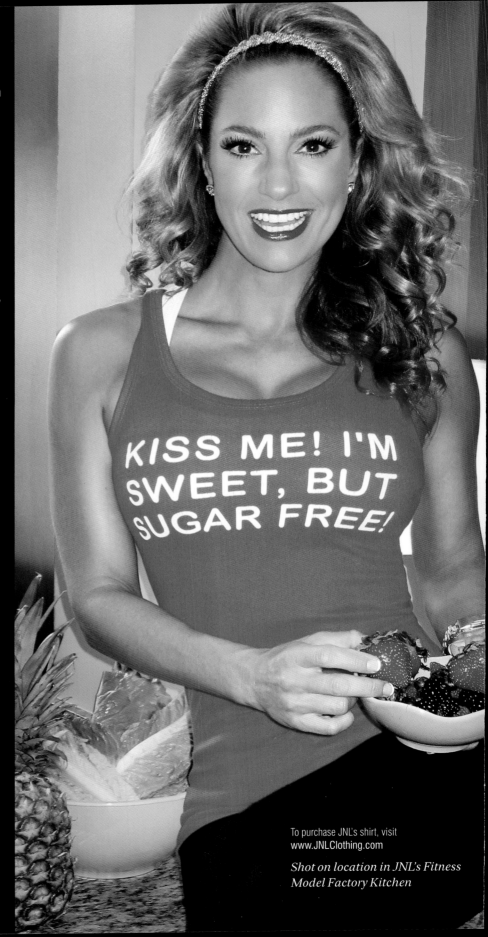

Fun, Fit Foodies, rejoice! YES, there is always room for dessert in our style of healthy living. When your sweet tooth strikes, have no fear — just flip to this chapter!

Welcome to one of my all-time favorite chapters; the one dedicated and devoted to desserts! In order to keep your sanity, and enjoy the decadent aspects of true celebratory eating, we must tantalize our taste buds with the different textures and sensations of dessert.

12. DESSERTS

To purchase JNL's shirt, visit
www.JNLClothing.com

Shot on location in JNL's Fitness Model Factory Kitchen

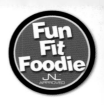

Chocolate Pound Cake with Cappuccino Pudding

This pudding gets its creamy texture by using silken tofu. Tofu is low in saturated fat, low in sodium and high in fiber.

INGREDIENTS:

- 2 cups silken tofu
- ½ cup extra dark chocolate, melted
- 1 tbsp dry instant coffee or espresso
- 1 tsp boiling water
- ½ cup low-fat sour cream
- ¼ cup honey (or to taste)
- 1 tsp vanilla extract
- ½ tsp ground cinnamon
- 1 fat-free chocolate pound cake
- Strawberries (optional)
- Toasted slivered almonds (optional)

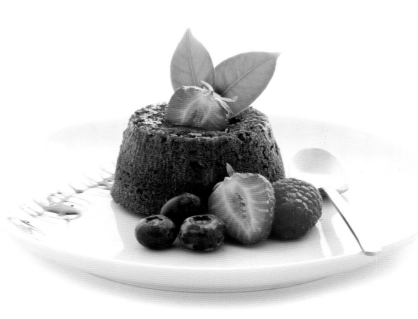

DIRECTIONS:

1. Drain the tofu and pulse in food processor until smooth. Melt the dark chocolate and add to tofu. Stir the instant coffee with boiling water and blend into the tofu. Add the sour cream, honey, vanilla and cinnamon; blend until creamy.

2. Slice pound cake into 8 portions and place on serving dishes. Add a large dollop of the pudding mixture. Garnish with strawberries and almonds (if using). Serves 8.

NUTRIENTS PER SERVING

Calories: 270

Total Fat: 8g
Saturated Fat: 4.5g
Cholesterol: 5mg
Sodium: 190mg
Total Carbohydrate: 44g
Dietary Fiber: 1g
Sugars: 28g
Protein: 7g

% Daily Value
Vit A: 0%   Vit C: 0%
Calcium: 6%   Iron: 10%

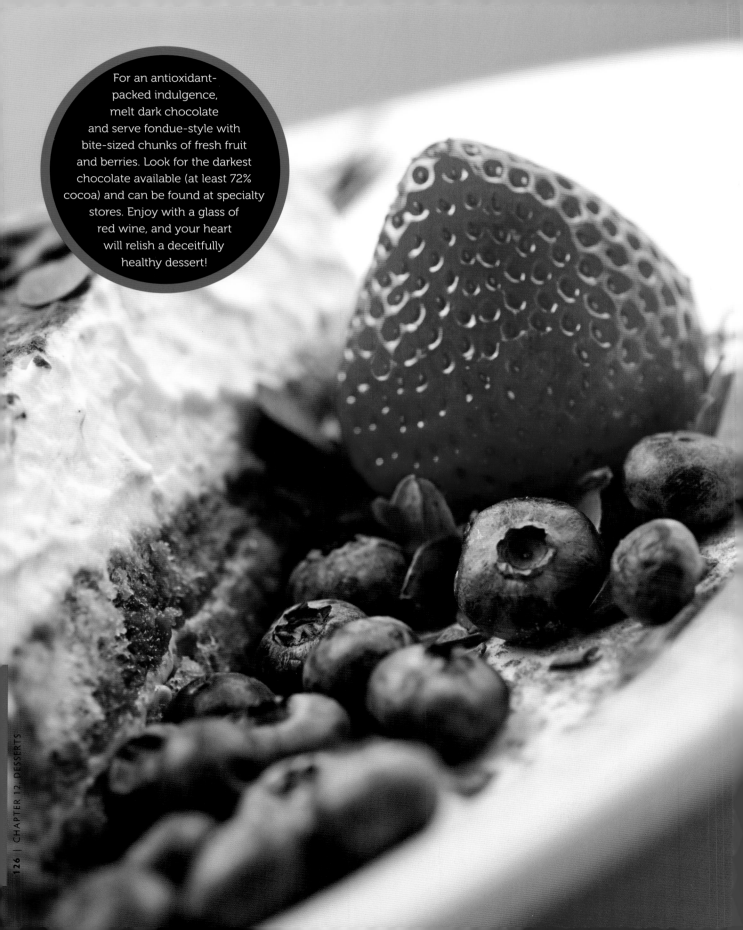

For an antioxidant-packed indulgence, melt dark chocolate and serve fondue-style with bite-sized chunks of fresh fruit and berries. Look for the darkest chocolate available (at least 72% cocoa) and can be found at specialty stores. Enjoy with a glass of red wine, and your heart will relish a deceitfully healthy dessert!

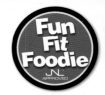

Sicilian Tiramisu

Inspired by my mom's tiramisu recipe, but with a healthier twist. I've trimmed extra fat by using ricotta instead of mascarpone. I added a punch of antioxidants and vitamin C with the berries! Add some espresso and ladyfingers, and I'm in heaven! Portion control is key so this is a great recipe for a large family gathering or a celebration.

INGREDIENTS:

- 2 cups fat-free ricotta cheese
- 2 tbsp cocoa powder
- 5 tsp instant espresso powder or instant strong coffee powder
- 1 tsp honey
- 1 tsp vanilla extract
- 1 tsp almond extract
- 10 soft ladyfingers
- 1 ½ cups fat-free chocolate pudding
- 2 cups sliced fresh strawberries
- Light real whipped cream
- Toasted slivered almonds

DIRECTIONS:

1. Blend the ricotta cheese with the cocoa powder, instant coffee, honey, vanilla extract and almond extract. Set aside.

2. Layer the ingredients into a 9-inch square glass pan or serving dish in the following order: ladyfingers, ricotta mixture, chocolate pudding and strawberries. Top with an even layer of whipped cream. Garnish with additional strawberries and toasted almonds. Serves 12.

JNL'S FUN, FIT FOODIE TIP: Your heart needs chocolate! Rejoice, Fun Fit Foodies, chocolate is healthy for you! In fact, it is so healthy that your heart actually loves you back for eating it. Studies have linked eating a chunk of extra dark chocolate with lower blood pressure, lower levels of bad cholesterol and reduced risk of stroke and heart attack. But more isn't necessarily better, so try to eat a chunk every other day. What makes chocolate so healthy for you? It's the flavonoids! Higher amounts in dark chocolate make it the top pick. Flavonoids keep blood vessels flexible and reduce the clumping of platelets that block heart arteries.

The power of cocoa is unquestionable. Cocoa has been shown to:
• Decrease blood pressure • Improve circulation • Lower death rate from heart disease • Improve function of endothelial cells that line blood vessels • Defend against destructive molecules called free radicals, which trigger cancer, heart disease, and stroke • Improve digestion and stimulate kidneys • Be beneficial to patients with anemia, kidney stones, and poor appetite

NUTRIENTS PER SERVING

Calories: 210

Total Fat: 4.5g
Saturated Fat: 2g
Cholesterol: 60mg
Sodium: 170mg
Total Carbohydrate: 32g
Dietary Fiber: 2g
Sugars: 17g
Protein: 9g

% Daily Value
Vit A: 2% Vit C: 40%
Calcium: 15% Iron: 8%

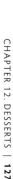

Angelic Mixed Berry Trifle

Egg white-based angel food cake makes a fluffy layer is this light and fruity classic dessert.

INGREDIENTS:

- 2 cups thick, low-fat vanilla yogurt (such as Greek yogurt)
- 1 ½ tsp finely grated orange zest
- 4 cups angel food cake, cubed
- 4 cups fresh or frozen thawed, drained, mixed berries
- 2 tbsp honey

DIRECTIONS:

1. Stir the yogurt with the orange zest. Place half the cubed cake in an 8-cup, glass serving bowl. Toss berries with honey; spread half of the berries over the cake cubes. Top with half of the yogurt mixture. Repeat the layers once.

2. Let stand, in refrigerator for at least 1 hour. Garnish with orange peel twists or additional berries. Makes 6 servings.

Grapefruit Tart

Deliciously tart with a creamy vanilla pudding filling on tender pound cake. So easy yet so elegant!

INGREDIENTS:

- 2 pink grapefruits
- 1 orange
- ½ cup fat-free, sugar-free vanilla pudding
- 8 pre-baked sponge cake shells

DIRECTIONS:

1. Using a sharp knife, peel rind and white pith from grapefruits and orange. Cut into sections and set in a strainer to drain.

2. Spread a small amount vanilla pudding over a sponge cake shell. Arrange drained grapefruit and orange sections over pudding. Serve immediately. Serves 8.

NUTRIENTS PER SERVING

Calories: 160

Total Fat: 2g	
Saturated Fat: 0.5g	
Cholesterol: 5mg	
Sodium: 210mg	
Total Carbohydrate: 34g	
Dietary Fiber: 4g	
Sugars: 18g	
Protein: 6g	

% Daily Value
Vit A: 2% Vit C: 15%
Calcium: 20% Iron: 2%

NUTRIENTS PER SERVING

Calories: 250

Total Fat: 2g	
Saturated Fat: 0g	
Cholesterol: 55mg	
Sodium: 870mg	
Total Carbohydrate: 57g	
Dietary Fiber: 2g	
Sugars: 27g	
Protein: 4g	

% Daily Value
Vit A: 0% Vit C: 50%
Calcium: 8% Iron: 8%

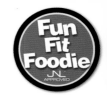

Roasted Pears and Peaches with Honey-Yogurt Sauce

While pears and peaches are loaded with fiber, walnuts are loaded with Omega-3 fat, and blueberries are an antioxidant powerhouse. It would be sinful NOT to eat this dessert, because it is just so good for you!

INGREDIENTS:

- 1 cup low-fat vanilla yogurt
- 2 tbsp honey
- 1 tbsp fresh lemon juice
- 1 tbsp coconut oil (approx.)
- 1 pint of blueberries
- ¼ cup chopped fresh mint
- 4 ripe pears, halved and cored
- 4 ripe peaches, peeled, halved and pitted
- 2 tbsp chopped toasted walnuts
- 2 tbsp unsweetened coconut flakes

JNL'S FUN, FIT FOODIE TIP: There is one sweetener you can feel guilt-free about: HONEY! Honey is a delish disease fighter. Now, you can feel good about putting your sweet tooth first. Put honey on the top of your sweet condiment list, as it's rich in cancer-fighting polyphenols. It's an immune-boosting sweetener which can be drizzled right onto fruit, spooned over crisp, whole-grain breads, or even dolloped right into a cup of plain yogurt!

DIRECTIONS:

1. Preheat the oven to 300°F. Whisk the yogurt with the honey, lemon juice and coconut oil in a small bowl. Toss blueberries with mint in a second bowl. Reserve in the fridge until ready to serve.

2. Lightly brush pears and peaches with additional coconut oil; transfer to a rimmed baking sheet and roast until tender. Chop into bite-sized pieces; toss with reserved blueberries and mint.

3. Evenly divide among eight serving dishes; drizzle with the honey sauce. Garnish with walnuts and coconut. Serves 8.

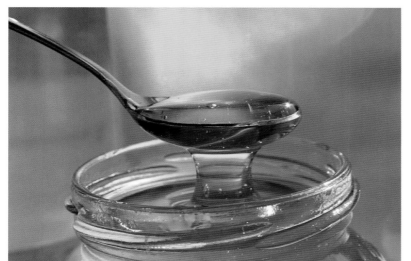

NUTRIENTS PER SERVING

Calories: 170
Total Fat: 5g
Saturated Fat: 3g
Cholesterol: 0mg
Sodium: 20mg
Total Carbohydrate: 33g
Dietary Fiber: 5g
Sugars: 24g
Protein: 3g

% Daily Value
Vit A: 0%   Vit C: 20%
Calcium: 8%   Iron: 2%

Honey & Wine Poached Pears

Red wine and honey are used to poach ripe pears and then simmered until thick and saucy. The red wine syrup can be stored in an airtight container for up to 1 week and drizzled over fruit, yogurt or waffles. For a sweet and savory combination, sprinkle pears with a little crumbled blue cheese and toasted walnuts before drizzling with syrup.

INGREDIENTS:

- 1 lemon
- 2 cups light bodied red wine
- 2 cups cranberry juice
- ½ cup honey
- 1 cinnamon stick
- 1 vanilla bean pod, scraped (reserve pod)
- 4 ripe Bosc pears, peeled, halved and cored

DIRECTIONS:

1. Use a vegetable peeler to remove two thin strips of peel from the lemon. Juice ½ of the lemon. (Reserve the remaining lemon half for another use.)

2. Combine the wine, cranberry juice, honey, lemon juice, lemon peel, cinnamon stick, vanilla bean scrapings and pod to a deep skillet. Bring poaching liquid to a boil over high heat and simmer for 5 to 6 minutes to let flavors develop. Add pears, and reduce the heat to medium-low. Simmer, partially covered and turning the pears often, for 15 to 20 minutes or until tender.

3. Use a slotted spoon to remove the pears from the poaching liquid. Increase the heat to medium. Simmer the liquid for 15 minutes or until it is reduced and thickened to a syrup. Taste and adjust for sweetness or tang by adding a little honey or lemon juice. Strain the poaching liquid. Arrange pear halves on dessert plates and drizzle with a little of the syrup to garnish. Serves 4.

JNL'S FUN, FIT FOODIE TIP: When I travelled in Asia, I discovered that dessert was a staple course at both lunch and dinner. However, the desserts were always a piece of fruit, usually a slice of watermelon or an orange wedge. I enjoyed seeing how they made it a point to finish off a meal with a sweet, juicy piece of fruit, banishing the myth that all desserts must be full of fat or empty calories.

NUTRIENTS PER SERVING

Calories: 240	
Total Fat: 0g	
Saturated Fat: 0g	
Cholesterol: 0mg	
Sodium: 10mg	
Total Carbohydrate: 53g	
Dietary Fiber: 4g	
Sugars: 42g	
Protein: 1g	

% Daily Value
Vit A: 2%   Vit C: 40%
Calcium: 4%   Iron: 4%

Walnut and Raisin Whole-Wheat Oatmeal Cookies

This is my husband's all-time favorite cookie! It's the perfect balance of not-too-sweet chewiness combined with the heart-healthy benefits of oatmeal. Enjoy this with a cup of green tea, and you will be enjoying an antioxidant, fiber-rich desert that's too good to be bad for you!

INGREDIENTS:

- 1 cup whole-wheat flour
- 1 tsp ground cinnamon
- 1 tsp baking powder
- ½ tsp baking soda
- ½ tsp salt
- 1 cup packed light brown sugar (or Splenda brown sugar substitute)
- ¼ cup unsweetened applesauce
- 2 egg whites
- 2 tbsp softened unsalted butter
- 1 ½ tsp vanilla
- 1 ⅓ cups uncooked large flake rolled oats
- ½ cup chopped walnuts
- ½ cup raisins (sultana or golden)

JNL'S FUN, FIT FOODIE TIP: Use the uncooked large flake (or old-fashioned) oatmeal; it's much healthier for you, since it's less processed. Remember, the quicker food is to cook, the more processing the food has undergone.

DIRECTIONS:

1. Preheat the oven to 375 F. Lightly coat cookie sheets with nonstick cooking spray. Stir the flour with the cinnamon, baking powder, baking soda and salt in medium bowl until combined.

2. Blend the brown sugar, applesauce, egg whites, butter and vanilla in large bowl until well-combined. Add the flour mixture; mix well. Stir in the oats, walnuts and raisins.

3. Drop by rounded spoonfuls of the cookie dough, 1 ½-inch apart, onto the prepared cookie sheets. Bake for 15 minutes, or until crispy brown on the bottoms. Cool on a wire rack. Makes about 3 ½ dozen cookies.

NUTRIENTS PER SERVING
(1 cookie)

Calories: 60

Total Fat: 1.5g	
Saturated Fat: 0.5g	
Cholesterol: 1mg	
Sodium: 50mg	
Total Carbohydrate: 10g	
Dietary Fiber: 1g	
Sugars: 5g	
Protein: 1g	

% Daily Value
Vit A: 0%   Vit C: 0%
Calcium: 0%   Iron: 2%

"Crazy Good" Coconut Cookies

They sound sinful but they are not. They are actually great for you, because they are low in sugar, high in fiber from the oats and the flax seeds add texture and essential fatty acids. What a great, guilt-free treat! Add a fat-free, snack-size cottage cheese and you are set until dinner.

INGREDIENTS:

- 3 tbsp warm water
- 1 tbsp honey
- 1 cup unsweetened flaked coconut
- 1 whole egg
- 1 tsp coconut oil
- 1 cup large flake rolled oats
- ¼ cup flax seeds

DIRECTIONS:

1. Preheat the oven to 400°F. Mix the warm water with the honey together until well combined; add the coconut flakes. Beat in the egg until well-combined. Stir in the oats and flaxseeds.

2. Grease a cookie sheet with the coconut oil. Form into balls and drop by spoonfuls on the prepared cookie sheet. Bake for 12 to 15 minutes. Makes about 1 dozen cookies.

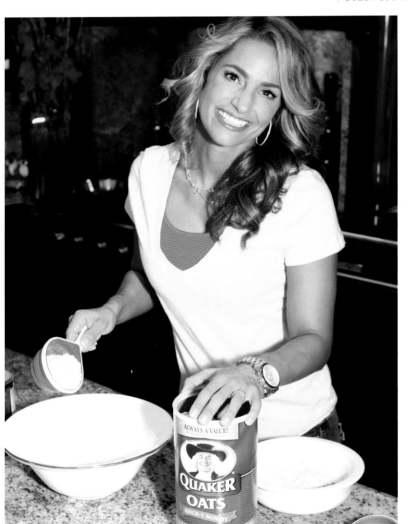

NUTRIENTS PER SERVING	
(1 cookie)	
Calories: 120	
Total Fat: 7g	
Saturated Fat: 4.5g	
Cholesterol: 15mg	
Sodium: 9mg	
Total Carbohydrate: 10g	
Dietary Fiber: 3g	
Sugars: 2g	
Protein: 3g	

% Daily Value
Vit A: 0%   Vit C: 0%
Calcium: 2%   Iron: 4%

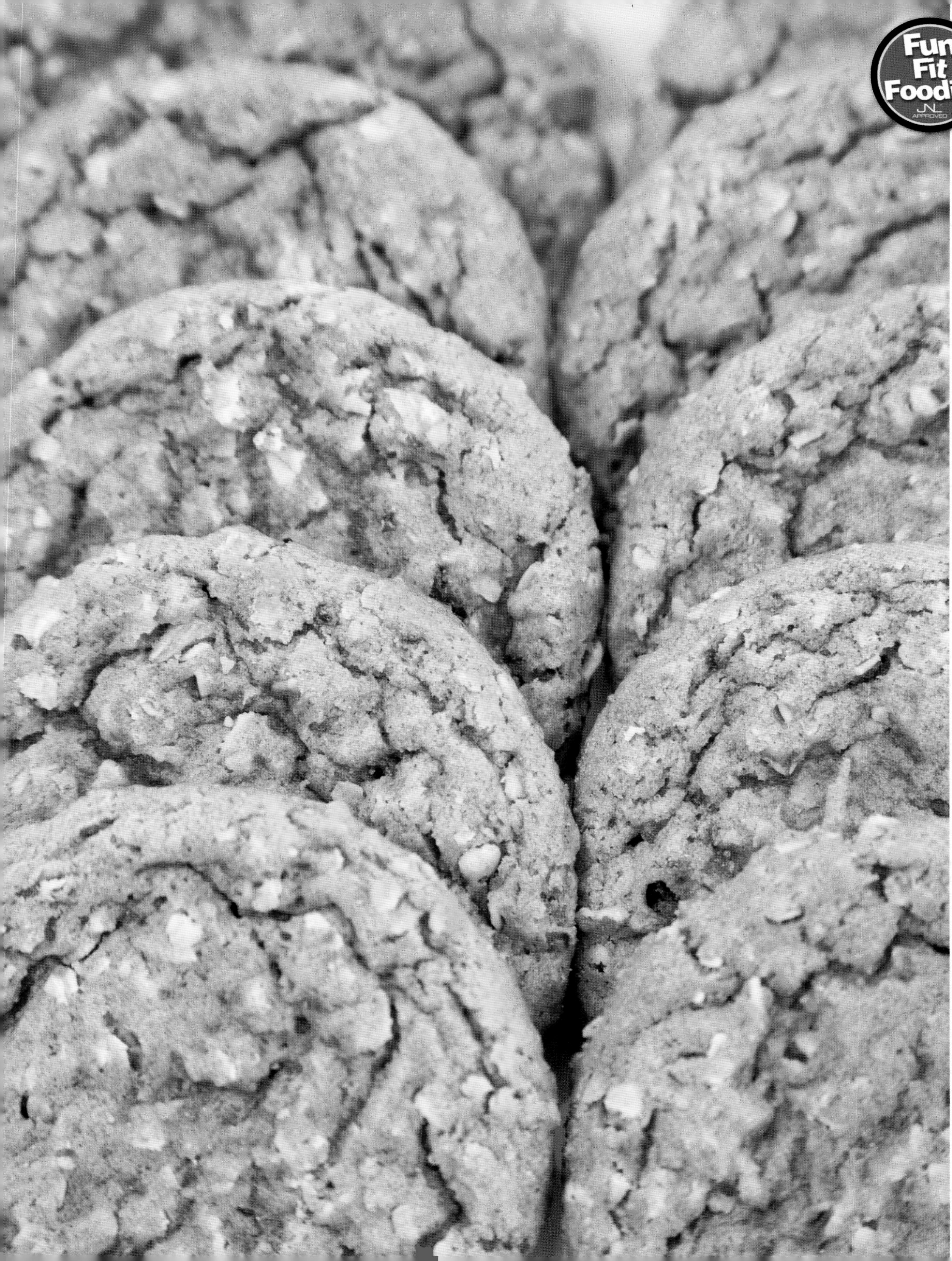

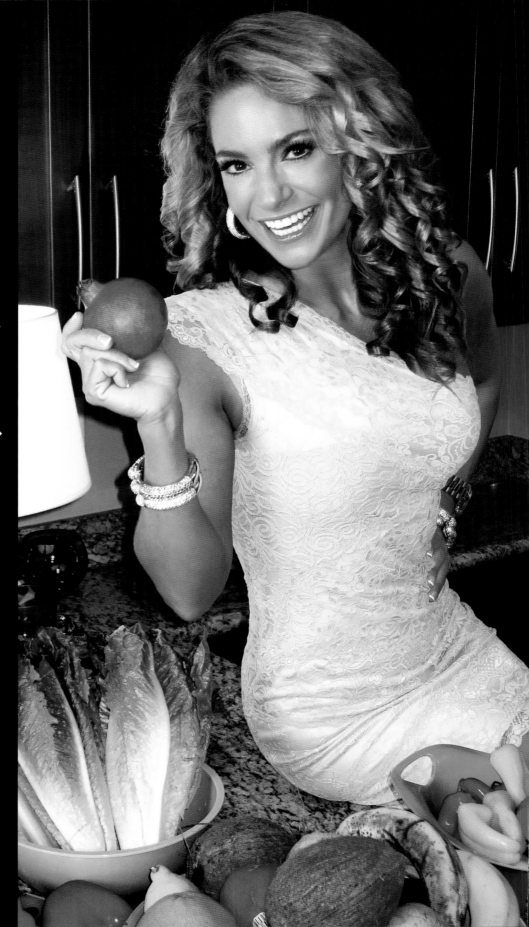

Cheers to the special time of the season where we spend time with our friends and family over hearty, home-cooked meals. The Holiday Feasts Chapter will help you create heartwarming meals, without making you pack on a good 15 pounds to fight off in the New Year!

I have taken classic holiday recipes and have tweaked them to make them as healthy as I could. Enjoy!

Fitness Model Factory Kitchen ▸

13. HOLIDAY FEASTS

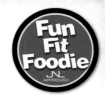

Healthy Green Bean Casserole

My sons Jaden and Dylan love to help me prepare the beans by snapping them in half, and this is one of their favorite sides. This is not the no-mess, super-easy recipe of yore, but it is low in fat and high in flavor. To go one step further, substitute ½ pound fresh green beans for frozen. Simply snap them into 1-inch lengths. Then blanch the beans for 1 to 2 minutes in boiling water, refresh under cold water and spread in the baking dish.

INGREDIENTS:

Topping

- ½ tsp canola oil
- 1 large onion, thinly sliced
- ½ cup fresh whole-wheat breadcrumbs

Casserole

- 2 cups skim milk
- 6 black peppercorns
- 1 bay leaf
- JAT grated nutmeg
- ½ tsp canola oil
- 1 small onion, finely chopped
- 3 cups sliced mushrooms (about ½ lb)
- 1 clove garlic, finely chopped
- ¼ cup all-purpose flour
- ¼ cup low-fat sour cream
- ½ tsp freshly ground pepper
- JAT sea salt
- 2 cups frozen green beans (about 9 oz)

DIRECTIONS:

1. Topping: Heat the oil in a large nonstick skillet set over low heat. Add the onion and cook, stirring occasionally, until very tender and golden, about 30 minutes. Set aside. Meanwhile, preheat the oven to 350°F. Spread breadcrumbs on a baking sheet. Bake, stirring once, for 6 to 10 minutes or until lightly browned. Set aside.

2. Casserole: Heat the milk with the peppercorns, bay leaf and nutmeg in a saucepan set over medium heat until steaming. Remove from the heat and let stand for 5 minutes to infuse the flavor. Strain into a measuring cup. (Discard peppercorns and bay leaf.)

3. Meanwhile, heat the oil in a large saucepan over medium heat. Add the onion and cook, stirring often, for 3 to 4 minutes or until golden. Add the mushrooms and garlic and cook, stirring, for 3 to 4 minutes or until tender.

4. Sprinkle the flour over the vegetables and cook, stirring, for 1 minute. Slowly pour in the infused milk, whisking constantly. Bring to a boil, stirring constantly. Reduce the heat to low and cook, stirring, for 1 minute or until thickened. Remove from the heat; whisk in the sour cream, pepper and salt.

5. Preheat oven to 425°F. Spread the green beans evenly over the bottom of a shallow 2-quart baking dish; pour the sauce evenly over the top. Toss the reserved onions with the toasted breadcrumbs in a small bowl and scatter over the beans. Bake until bubbling, 15 to 25 minutes. Serves 4 (recipe doubles easily).

NUTRIENTS PER SERVING

Calories: 180
Total Fat: 4g
Saturated Fat: 1.5g
Cholesterol: 10mg
Sodium: 700mg
Total Carbohydrate: 29g
Dietary Fiber: 4g
Sugars: 11g
Protein: 10g

% Daily Value
Vit A: 0%   Vit C: 15%
Calcium: 25%   Iron: 8%
Excellent source of riboflavin, vitamin D and selenium.

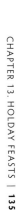

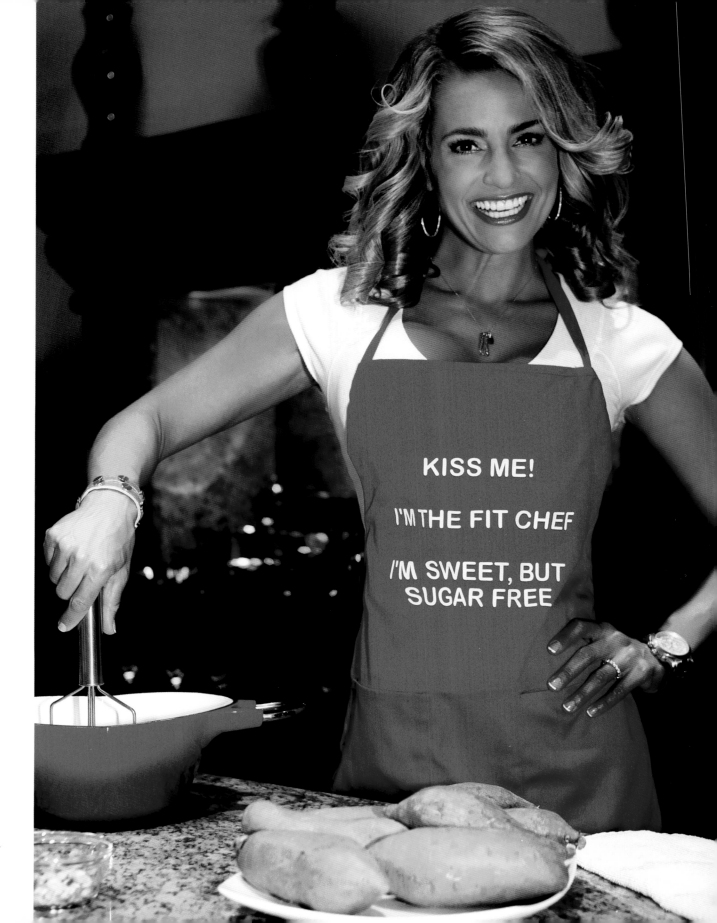

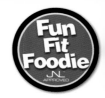

Healthy Sweet Potato Casserole

My husband loves this one, it's so rich and creamy and sweet, that it tastes like a dessert!

INGREDIENTS:

- 1 lb sweet potatoes, peeled and cut into ½-inch pieces
- ½ cup skim milk
- 2 eggs, beaten
- 2 tbsp honey
- 1 tsp vanilla extract
- JAT sea salt and freshly ground black pepper
- ¼ cup brown sugar
- ¼ cup chopped pecans
- 2 tbsp all-purpose flour
- 1 tbsp melted unsalted butter

DIRECTIONS:

1. Preheat the oven to 400°F. Place the sweet potatoes in a steamer basket set over boiling water. Cover and steam for 10 minutes or until tender. Remove from the steamer basket and mash until smooth. Cool slightly.

2. Stir sweet potatoes with the milk, eggs, honey and vanilla until well-combined. Season with salt and pepper. Spread into a lightly greased, 9-inch baking pan.

3. Toss the sugar with the pecans, flour and butter until crumbly. Sprinkle evenly over the sweet potato mixture. Bake for 30 minutes or until bubbly and browned. Serves 6.

NUTRIENTS PER SERVING

Calories: 170

Total Fat: 5g	
Saturated Fat: 1.5g	
Cholesterol: 5mg	
Sodium: 30mg	
Total Carbohydrate: 28g	
Dietary Fiber: 2g	
Sugars: 18g	
Protein: 2g	

% Daily Value
Vit A: 35%   Vit C: 15%
Calcium: 6%   Iron: 4%
Excellent source of manganese.

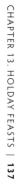

Roast Turkey with Champagne-Infused Apricot & Cran-Apple Stuffing

So darn good, it's hard to believe it's actually healthy for you! With a kick of pink champagne, the cran-apple and apricot stuffing is sure to be moist!

INGREDIENTS:

- 2 tbsp unsalted butter or olive oil
- 1 cup finely chopped onion
- 2 cloves garlic, minced
- 1 ½ cups low sodium chicken broth
- 1 ½ cups pink champagne
- 6 cups whole-wheat bread, torn into large pieces (day-old baguette preferred)
- ¾ cup dried apricots, chopped
- ½ cup dried cranberries, chopped
- ¾ cup tart apples such as Granny Smith, cut into bite-sized chunks
- 3 tbsp fresh rosemary, minced
- 3 tbsp fresh thyme, minced
- 2 tsp freshly ground black pepper, divided
- 1 whole turkey (about 14 lb), thawed if necessary

DIRECTIONS:

1. Melt the butter in a small saucepan set over medium heat. Add the onion and garlic and sauté until translucent. Stir in the broth and champagne; bring to a boil and remove from the heat. Meanwhile, arrange the bread in a large bowl. Pour the broth mixture over the bread. Stir to make sure the bread is evenly soaked. Let stand for 15 minutes or until cool enough to handle.

2. Squeeze the bread with your hands, breaking it up. Add the apricots, cranberries, apples, rosemary, thyme, and half of the pepper. Work the mixture with your hands until well blended.

3. Preheat the oven to 325°F (160°C). Remove the neck and giblets from the turkey and set aside for gravy (if desired). Rub the turkey inside and out with the remaining pepper. Fill the body and neck cavities loosely with the stuffing. Fasten the flaps with turkey skewers. Tie the legs together at the bottom using kitchen twine.

4. Place the turkey, breast-side-up, on a rack in a roasting pan. Roast, basting often with pan drippings, for about 3 hours (or 12 to 15 minutes per pound) or until an instant-read thermometer registers 165°F when inserted into the stuffing and thickest part of the breast and thigh without touching the bone. (Once the breast is golden, tent the turkey loosely with aluminum foil to prevent over-browning). Tent the turkey with foil and let stand for 20 minutes before carving. Serves 12 with leftovers.

NUTRIENTS PER SERVING

Calories: 440

Total Fat: 18g	
Saturated Fat: 6g	
Cholesterol: 140mg	
Sodium: 220mg	
Total Carbohydrate: 15g	
Dietary Fiber: 2g	
Sugars: 6g	
Protein: 49g	

% Daily Value
Vit A: 2%   Vit C: 2%
Calcium: 6%   Iron: 20%
Excellent source of niacin, vitamin B6, selenium, and zinc.

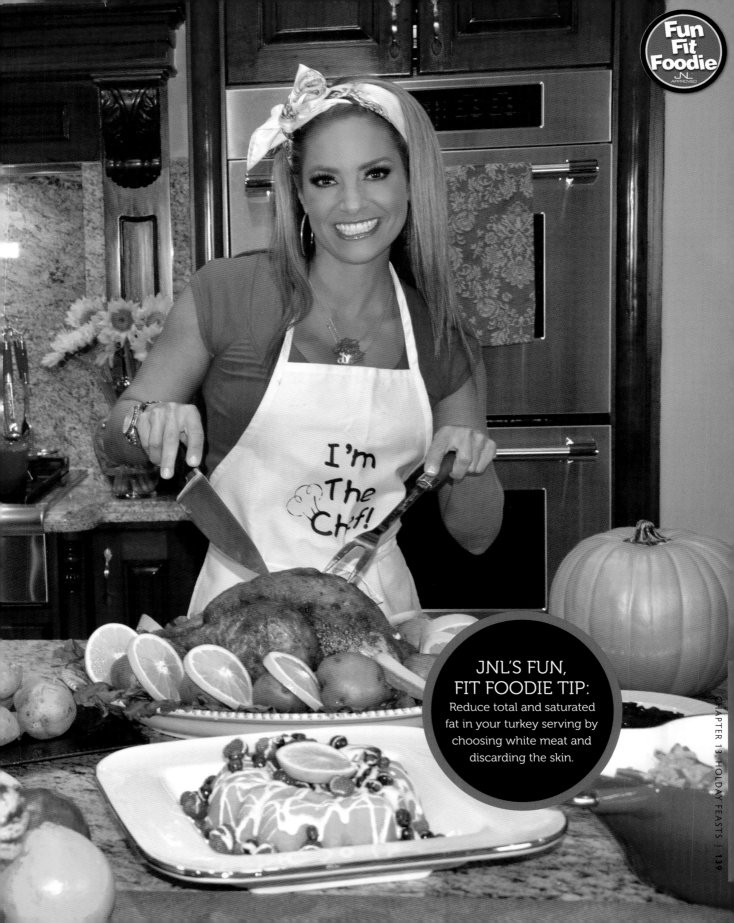

Fun Fit Foodie
JNL APPROVED

JNL'S FUN, FIT FOODIE TIP: Reduce total and saturated fat in your turkey serving by choosing white meat and discarding the skin.

Lower Fat Pumpkin Pie

It's too bad we only eat pumpkin pie at holidays! Pumpkin is super high in Beta-carotene, so dig in and enjoy.

INGREDIENTS:

- 1 can (15 oz) pure puréed pumpkin
- 1 can (14 oz) fat-free sweetened condensed milk
- ½ cup liquid egg substitute
- ½ tsp salt
- ½ tsp ground cinnamon
- ½ tsp ground nutmeg
- ½ tsp ground ginger
- 1 (9-inch) unbaked pie shell

DIRECTIONS:

1. Preheat the oven to 425°F.

2. Whisk the pumpkin with the condensed milk, egg substitute, salt, cinnamon, nutmeg and ginger in a large mixing bowl until smooth. Pour into the pie shell.

3. Bake for 15 minutes. Reduce the temperature to 350°F and bake for 25 to 30 minutes or until a knife inserted near the center comes out clean. Cool completely on a wire rack. Store leftover pie in the refrigerator. Serves 8.

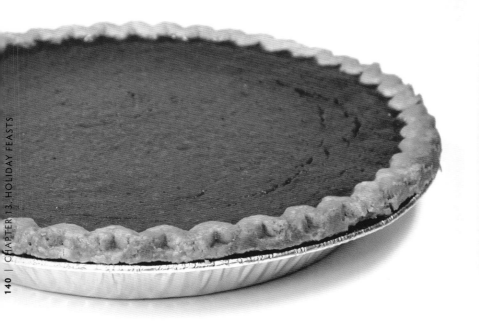

NUTRIENTS PER SERVING

Calories: 290

Total Fat: 8g	
Saturated Fat: 2g	
Cholesterol: 5mg	
Sodium: 320mg	
Total Carbohydrate: 46g	
Dietary Fiber: 3g	
Sugars: 32g	
Protein: 7g	

% Daily Value
Vit A: 140%   Vit C: 0%
Calcium: 15% Iron: 8%
Excellent source of riboflavin and vitamin B12.

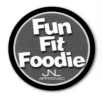

Stuffing with Fresh Cranberries

My personal favorite! Sautéing the vegetables in broth, allows me to cut out butter and fat from this satisfying side-dish.

INGREDIENTS:

- 1 cup low sodium chicken broth
- 1 cup chopped celery
- ½ cup chopped onion
- 4 cups whole wheat bread cubes
- 1 cup whole water chestnuts
- 1 cup chopped apple
- ½ cup cranberries, chopped
- ¼ cup chopped parsley
- 1 tsp dried tarragon
- ½ tsp paprika
- ⅛ tsp nutmeg

DIRECTIONS:

1. Preheat the oven to 350°F. Heat the chicken broth in a large skillet set over medium heat. Sauté the celery and onion in broth until tender. Remove from the heat and cool slightly.

2. Meanwhile, toss bread cubes with the water chestnuts, apple, cranberries, parsley, tarragon, paprika and nutmeg in a large bowl. Stir in the sautéed onion and celery as well as any remaining broth until well-combined.

3. Lightly coat a 2-quart baking dish with nonstick cooking spray. Spoon the stuffing mixture into the dish. Cover and bake for 20 minutes; uncover. Bake for 10 minutes or until golden. Serves 8.

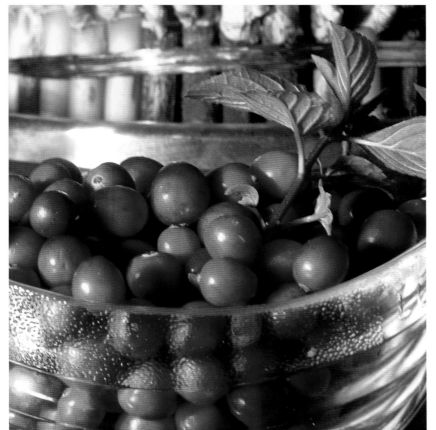

NUTRIENTS PER SERVING

Calories: 150

Total Fat: 2.5g	
Saturated Fat: 0g	
Cholesterol: 0mg	
Sodium: 250mg	
Total Carbohydrate: 29g	
Dietary Fiber: 5g	
Sugars: 7g	
Protein: 5g	

% Daily Value
Vit A: 2%   Vit C: 10%
Calcium: 4%   Iron: 8%

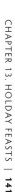

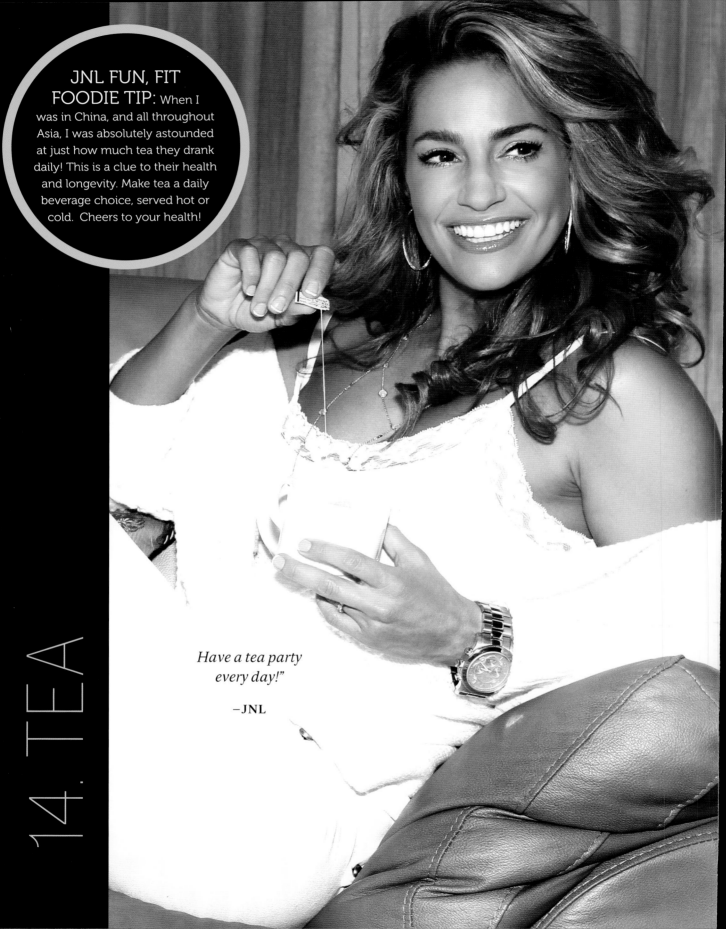

JNL FUN, FIT FOODIE TIP: When I was in China, and all throughout Asia, I was absolutely astounded at just how much tea they drank daily! This is a clue to their health and longevity. Make tea a daily beverage choice, served hot or cold. Cheers to your health!

Have a tea party every day!"

– JNL

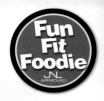

TEA HELPS YOU TO LOOK AND FEEL YOUNGER

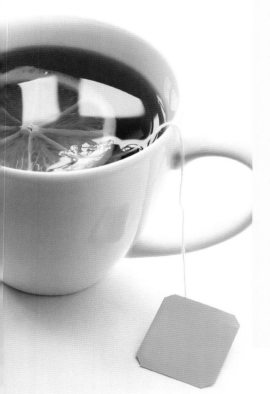

Yes, tea tastes great, and has been around for centuries. But there are SO many great reasons to drink it, that we all should at least sip one cup or two a day. Just take a look...

- Studies suggested that the high concentration of antioxidants in tea have an anti-aging effect. Antioxidants help to fight off free radicals, which cause cancer and disease. A cup or two a day will help keep the doctor away, thus helping you to have more energy and look better.

- Tea protects your bones. It's not just the milk added to tea that builds strong bones. One study that compared tea drinkers with non-drinkers, found that people who drank tea for 10 or more years had the strongest bones, even after adjusting for age, body weight, exercise, smoking and other risk factors. The authors suggest that this may be the work of tea's many beneficial phytochemicals.

- Tea strengthens your immune system. Drinking tea may help your body's immune system fight off infection. It's been around and used medicinally for centuries, to help fortify one's body, from the inside out. Vitamin C in green tea helps to treat the flu and the common cold. Moreover, the polyphenols in tea have been shown to increase the number of white blood cells in our immune system.

- Tea protects against cancer. Polyphenols are the antioxidants found in tea that fight cancer.

- Tea keeps you "moist and juicy." Hot water is transformed from boring to bold with just one little tea bag, causing you to drink more because it tastes so good! Thus you are hydrating your body more, more often.

- Calorie-free satisfaction: Sip on a cup of tea if you want something that's satisfying and calorie-free.

- Tea revs up your fat-burning furnace! Got a slow metabolic rate? You can actually change that, one cup of tea at a time! Green tea speeds up your metabolism; just drink five cups per day.
Even though researchers can't quite agree on every aspect, I'm sold on the fact that a few cups a day will help to protect me from heart disease, stroke, cancer, and more.

SO WHAT IS THE MAGIC IN TEA THAT MAKES IT SO POWERFUL?

Tea contains antioxidants, which fight off the free radicals in the body, and help keep them from harming your healthy cells. Tea is FULL of these antioxidants, in particular catechins, polyphenols, and flavonoids. This boils down to disease prevention. By drinking this antioxidant-rich brew daily, you are sending in disease fighters by the teacup full!

ASK JNL:
Which are the Best Teas?

Okay, so you are ready to drink more tea. Here are some answers to your common questions.

QUESTION: What teas have the most antioxidants, and are thus the healthiest?

ANSWER: Buy the best if you can! Higher quality teas may have more catechin antioxidants than lower quality teas.

QUESTION: What tea has the highest amount of antioxidants?

ANSWER: White tea.

QUESTION: If I had to choose between green and black tea, which one is better?

ANSWER: Since black tea goes through more processing, green tea has more catechin antioxidants.

QUESTION: Can I drink instant tea and get the same health benefits?

ANSWER: Instant or bottled teas have less polyphenol antioxidants than freshly brewed teas.

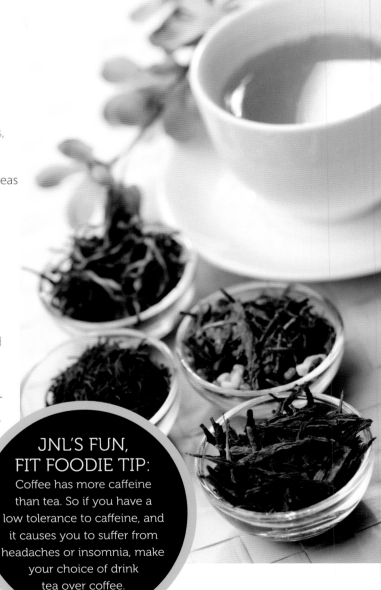

JNL'S FUN, FIT FOODIE TIP:
Coffee has more caffeine than tea. So if you have a low tolerance to caffeine, and it causes you to suffer from headaches or insomnia, make your choice of drink tea over coffee.

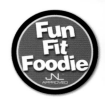

HERE IS MY FUN, FIT FOODIE LIST OF TEA TO DRINK FOR COMMON LIFESTYLE NEEDS:

CONDITION / PURPOSE	TEA
For Slimming	Oolong Tea
For High Blood Pressure	Banana Tea and Lotus Tea
For Coughs	White Radish Tea
For Itchy Throat But No Cough	Licorice Tea
For Dry Sore Throat	Honey Lemon Tea
For Flu	Lei Cha Tea
For Quenching Thirst & Mild Sunstroke	Cold Chrysanthemum Tea
For Restoring Energy	Ginseng Tea
For Relieving Stress	Rose Green Tea
For Reducing High Cholesterol & High Blood Pressure	Imperial Kuding Tea
For Helping With Weight Loss	Wild Bitter Tea

HERE ARE SOME OF MY FAVORITE TEAS!

White Tea

Green Tea

Black Tea

Chai Tea – try my Fun, Fit Foodie Favorite Decaf Chai Tea by Tazo®

Wu Long (Or Oolong) Tea

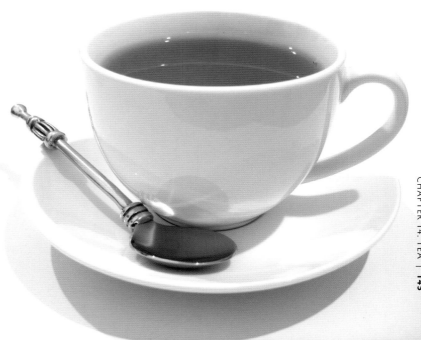

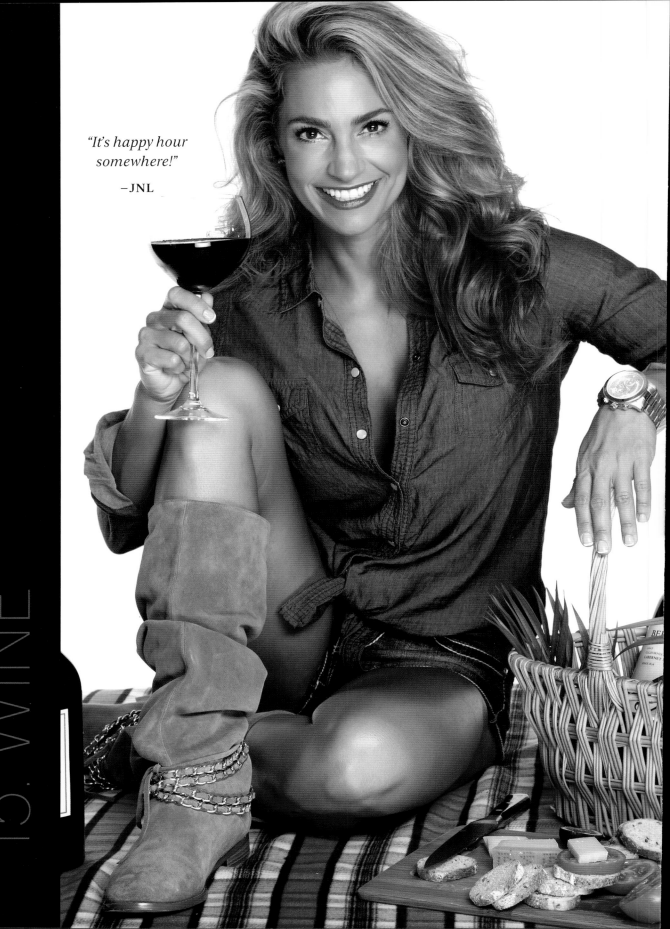

"It's happy hour somewhere!"

–JNL

15. WINE

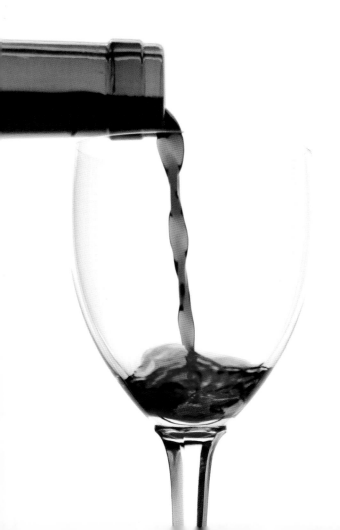

Being Italian, I grew up seeing my family enjoy red wine. Many fitness experts state that a glass of wine a day helps you actually to be healthier. My Italian grandparents always drank a small glass of red wine at lunch, and another at dinner. They both enjoyed long lives and were full of energy and stamina.

The Mediterranean diet is linked to many health benefits, and this includes the advantages of red wine! And as part of being a devout foodie, you've got to love a great glass of wine. So, in my Fun, Fit Foodie lifestyle, we embrace the heart-healthy benefits of a glass of wine a day.

WOW Health Benefits of Red Wine!

We all know from years and years of research that the leading experts agree that drinking a moderate amount of red wine can help lower cholesterol and prevent heart disease, tooth decay, and possibly even Alzheimer's disease.

I don't know if all of this is true, but I know for sure that I love to drink one glass of red wine a day, and that it really does help me to take the edge off the day, de-stress and relax. I used to feel a bit guilty about it, but with all the new research coming out about the health benefits of red wine, I'm feeling pretty good about enjoying this little daily pleasure.

Go Red!

It's true, some wines are healthier than others, and when in doubt, GO RED! Unfortunately for fans of white zinfandel, white wine does not deliver the same health benefits as a good glass of Merlot or a Cab!

RED WINE AND CARDIOVASCULAR HEALTH

True to the "Fun, Fit Foodie" philosophy, everything is fine in moderation, right? So then this also pertains to "the drink of the Greek gods" (or goddesses too!), red wine, right? In moderation, red wine has for a while now been regarded as good for the ol' ticker, as it is healthy for the heart.

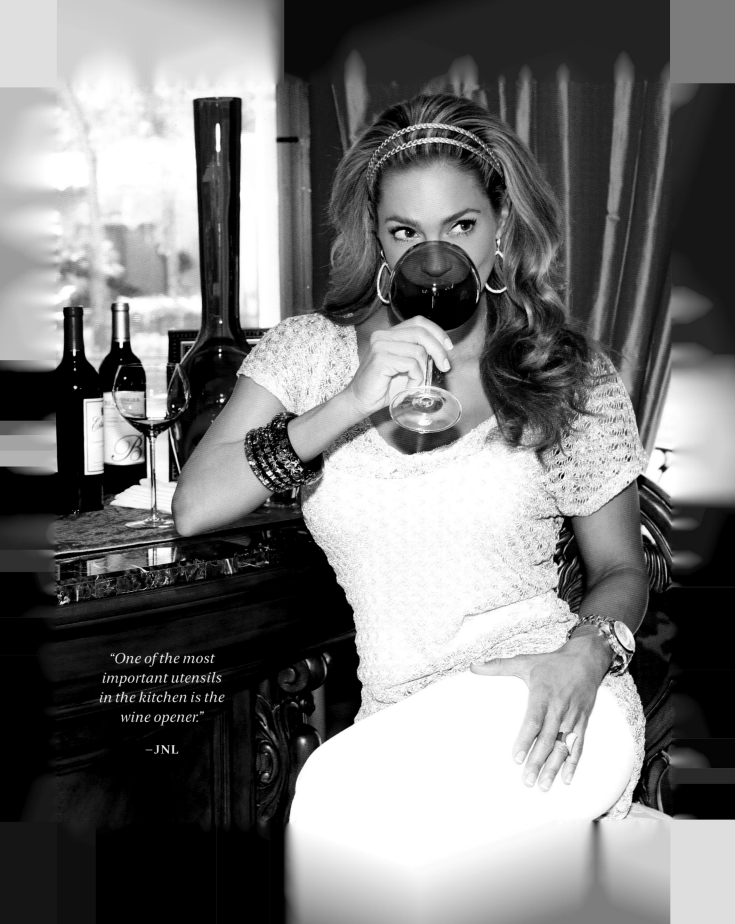

"One of the most important utensils in the kitchen is the wine opener."

–JNL

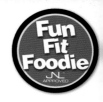

So what's the secret in red wine that's so darn good for us? The secret are antioxidants that actually just may aid in preventing the number one silent killer of women, which is heart disease. How is this done? The antioxidants found in red wine actually defend in damage of arteries while also raising levels of good cholesterol. Pretty cool, huh? So that's why all Fun, Fit Foodies say that the most important kitchen utensil is the wine opener!

"Nothing more excellent or valuable than wine was ever granted by the Gods to man."

—PLATO

FUN, FIT FOODIES LOVE RED WINE, AS RED WINE LOVES OUR HEARTS!

Listen, I love red wine, because red wine loves me and loves my heart. Again in moderation, the health benefits are immense. So cheers to a glass in honor of our heart health and increasing our antioxidant intake. And in great depth, the real secret ingredient in wine are flavonoids, which are powerful potent antioxidants that are in certain foods-from fruits to chocolate, and yes beer and even white wine. But what makes red wine the Queen of drinks, is her higher Resveratrol levels, which have been linked to prevention of damage of blood vessels. And if you have to lower your bad cholesterol, this is good news for you, as red wine has also been shown to do just that.

That's a lot of scientific jargon, so let me boil it down for you the Fun, Fit Foodie way:

"A glass of red wine a day keeps the doctor away!"

To be clear, drinking red wine in moderation will give you these health benefits. So don't go overboard! Guys, that's two glasses a day, and gals, that's one glass a day! Don't go over that amount, as too much alcohol can have many harmful effects on your body.

Antioxidants aren't the only substances in red wine that look promising. The alcohol in red wine also appears to be heart healthy. Learn more about what's known — and not known — about red wine and its possible heart-health benefits, and make sure that you "feed your heart" daily by getting in your glass of red wine.

So in closing, cheers to your health! Raise a glass a day in celebration of living the heart-healthy Fun, Fit Foodie way!

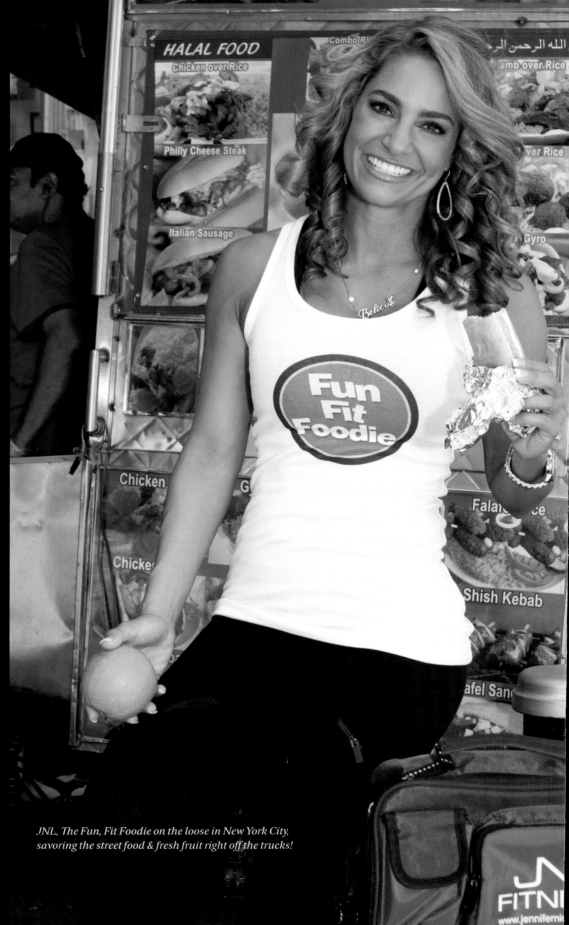

JNL, The Fun, Fit Foodie on the loose in New York City, savoring the street food & fresh fruit right off the trucks!

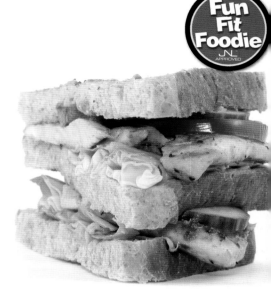

W e all work and have busy lives with overbooked schedules and demands that we cannot keep up with. Some days we simply don't have time to "juli-enne" red pepper, mince garlic and defrost chicken!

Let's face it, even though cooking and preparing meals does have nutri-tional benefits, we can't do it every day. So, when we are out in the real world, what do we eat? With my fail-proof list of do's and don'ts, and what to look for and what to avoid, eating out or eating on-the-go is a cinch!

FUN, FIT FOODIE EATING OUT GUIDELINES:

WHAT TO AVOID	WHAT TO LOOK FOR	WHAT TO DO
Fried foods; instead steam, poach or sauté foods in canola oil.	Baked or grilled meats.	Ask for grilled instead of fried.
Foods loaded with gravies or heavy sauces; ask for it on the side, if you've got to have it.	Low-sodium alternatives.	Always ask the chef to omit cheese, sour cream and soy sauce (they are loaded with unnecessary fats and/or sodium).
Sugary treats disguised as healthy foods (granola bars, "snack mix," breakfast bars, etc.)	Fresh vegetables and fruits.	
Colas and other sugared soft drinks that pack a whopping 200 calories per serving.	Low-fat, snack-size servings that are low in sugar. Read the nutritional facts on the label! You can't assume it is healthy even if the word "healthy" is part of the product's name.	Ask for water instead of the diet soda or cola that comes with your meal combo. It's better for you and you don't need those chemicals. Choose low-fat milk or skim milk instead of whole milk or half & half.
Sandwiches made with white bread.	Whole wheat bread or brown rice or other whole grains as a side.	Always choose whole wheat or whole grain bread when given a choice.
Mayonnaise, oil, butter, margarine.	Olive oil and flax seed oil.	Always ask for sauce or dressings on the side.

Learning how to healthfully eat on-the-go is part of mastering the Fun, Fit Foodie lifestyle. With the increasing amount of "healthy food" options which most fast food chains are now offering, there are no more excuses!

SUBWAY	• Any six inch sandwich on whole wheat bread from their "7 under 6" menu (forgo the cheese, mayonnaise, oil and salt, and load up on the veggies!) • Turkey Breast • Roasted Chicken Breast • Sweet Onion Chicken Teriyaki • Roast Beef • Tuna Salad made with low-fat mayonnaise
WENDY'S	• Southwest Chicken Caesar Salad • Mandarin Chicken Caesar Salad • Southwest Taco Salad (forgo sour cream) • Chicken BLT Salad • Grilled Chicken Sandwich (no mayo or cheese, top bun off, and opt for lettuce & tomato) • Grilled Chicken Wrap (no mayo or cheese, top bun off, and opt for lettuce & tomato) • Side Salad with Low-fat Honey mustard • Diet Lemonade or Bottled Water • Small Chili and Side Salad
MCDONALDS	• Southwest Salad with Grilled Chicken • Asian Salad with Grilled Chicken • Premium Bacon Ranch Salad with Grilled Chicken • Premium Caesar Salad with Chicken • Snack Size Fruit & Walnut Salad • Grilled Chicken Classic (no mayo or cheese, top bun off, and opt for lettuce & tomato) • Grilled Snack Wrap (ask for no cheese, add lettuce & tomato)

TACO BELL	• Soft Tacos • Steak or Chicken Al Fresco (no cheese, no sour cream or Guacamole; just made with lettuce and tomatoes) • Crunchy taco Fresco style • Beef or Chicken Soft Taco • Ranchero Chicken Soft Taco Fresco Style • Bean Burrito Fresco Style • Chicken Burrito Fresco Style • Steak Burrito Fresco Style
BURGER KING	• Chicken Caesar Salad • Shrimp Caesar Salad • Chicken Garden Salad • Shrimp Garden Salad • Plain hamburger (no mayonnaise; opt for lettuce and tomato instead) • Grilled chicken (no mayonnaise; opt for lettuce and tomato instead) • Veggie Burger

JNL'S FUN, FIT FOODIE TIP:
Toss the top bun of your sandwich, so you are only eating the bottom bun. This little Fun, Fit Foodie tip will help you to eat less carbs, yet still enjoy the sandwich.

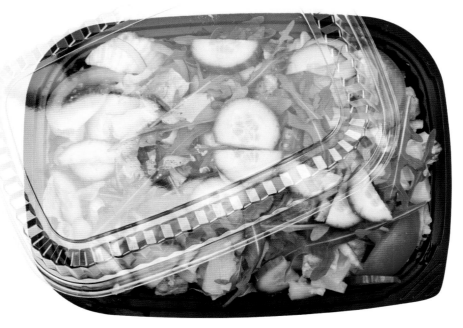

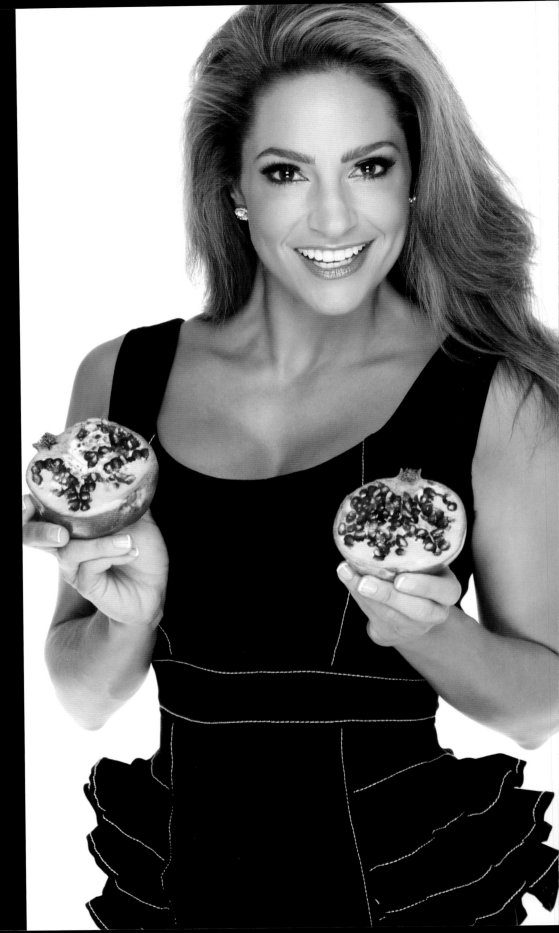

This chapter is dedicated to my Fun, Fit Foodies and your frequently asked questions.

If you have a question that's not addressed here, make sure you visit www.TheFunFitFoodie.com and email it to me.

Q JNL, as a Fun, Fit Foodie, do you allow for occasional Cheat Meals in your plan?

A Great question! As a professional in the fitness industry, I am often asked if I enjoy a cheat meal or a cheat day. My answer is based on wisdom, common sense, reason, and logic. If I have the mindset that I am starving myself from the get-go, I will not get results. I am eating to live, not living to eat. I don't designate a day of the week just to binge, or to eat whatever I want and however much of it I want! Instead, I am reasonable, balanced and focused with my food plan. Having two growing boys around all the time is great for my willpower. I am constantly bombarded with Oreos, mac & cheese, pizza, hot dogs, chicken nuggets and French fries. But instead of a "cheat meal" in which I could easily consume over 1,000 calories

(Fettuccini Alfredo, anyone?), I savor a "cheat bite." Sometimes the small nibble from my son's chocolate chip cookie is just as satisfying, if not more so, than eating the whole thing. I get to enjoy the small taste and the aroma of the cookie, without having to work out twice as hard to burn off all those extra calories I'd have taken in if I had eaten the whole cookie.

Taking "cheat bites" really helps when you are at dinner parties or work functions where everyone else is eating and you don't want to look or feel left out. Simply take your piece of key lime pie, eat one bite, and then leave the rest! Believe me, you will feel so good and proud of yourself when you are looking back at that plate with the rest of the uneaten pie you left behind, along with all the unnecessary calories that you saved by not eating the whole piece.

Q And what do you do if you ate that extra piece of pie or indulged a little too much?

A You simply keep your eye on the prize and pick up right where you left off!

Eat healthy again, admit that you can do better, exercise, and plan not to repeat the cycle.

Q JNL, I've heard you say that most high-end coffee drinks are really nothing but hot milkshakes, full of empty calories and sugar. What can I order at my local Starbucks that will give me my creamy coffee fix, thus allowing me to be a Fun, Fit Foodie, but without going overboard with the calories?

A I love Starbucks, too! And the great news is all you have to do is ask for the "Skinny" version of whatever is your favorite coffee drink. They will create a non-fat drink for you, made with sugar-free syrup and non-fat milk. According to Starbucks, this new coffee has at least 50 percent fewer calories than one made with regular syrup. The new 12-oz Café Latte has 90 calories, whereas the normal 12-oz white chocolate mocha latte has nearly 400 calories. So, the next time, you do not have to mention "non-fat and sugar free"; just telling your barista that you want a "skinny" latte will do.

Q: *I see that you get a lot of flavor to your stocks, stews, and pressure cooking recipes by cooking with red and white wine. Should I use cooking wine to cook with?*

A: Simple rule of thumb: Don't cook with anything that you wouldn't drink. Please don't use cooking wine to cook with, but a decent quality wine that would taste good with what you're cooking.

....

Q: *JNL, I'm so glad you endorse eating a chunk of chocolate a day, or every other day. What's your favorite kind, and what should we look for?*

A: Look for the darkest percentage you can get! I like Lindt, Godiva, and Dove. Aim for over 80% cacao.

Q: *JNL, what's your favorite wine?*

A: I'm a red wine girl, as it's got the more antioxidant bang per glass. I always opt for a full- bodied, robust cab. I like a wine to kiss me back when I sip it! The more body the better. I love any red wine from these labels:

- Shafer Vineyards
- Beaulieu Vineyard
- Mondavi
- Beringer
- Penfold's
- Grgich Hills
- Sterling Vineyards
- Pine Ridge
- Screaming Eagle
- Stag's Leap Wine Cellars
- Chateau St. Jean
- McManis
- Hogue
- Jardin
- Montes
- Concha Y Toro
- Columbia-Crest

The best way to learn about wine is to try a new bottle every week, to discover what your taste buds and palate prefer.

....

Q: *JNL, If I want to meet other Fun, Fit Foodies, see online cooking demos, and swap recipes, where should I go?*

A: One place! Visit www.TheFunFitFoodie.tv

"Life is too short to take your food so seriously. Once you stop counting calories, quit measuring out food, and call a halt to dieting, and just start eating the Fun, Fit Foodie way, you will have more fun, be more fit, and get in great shape!"

–JNL

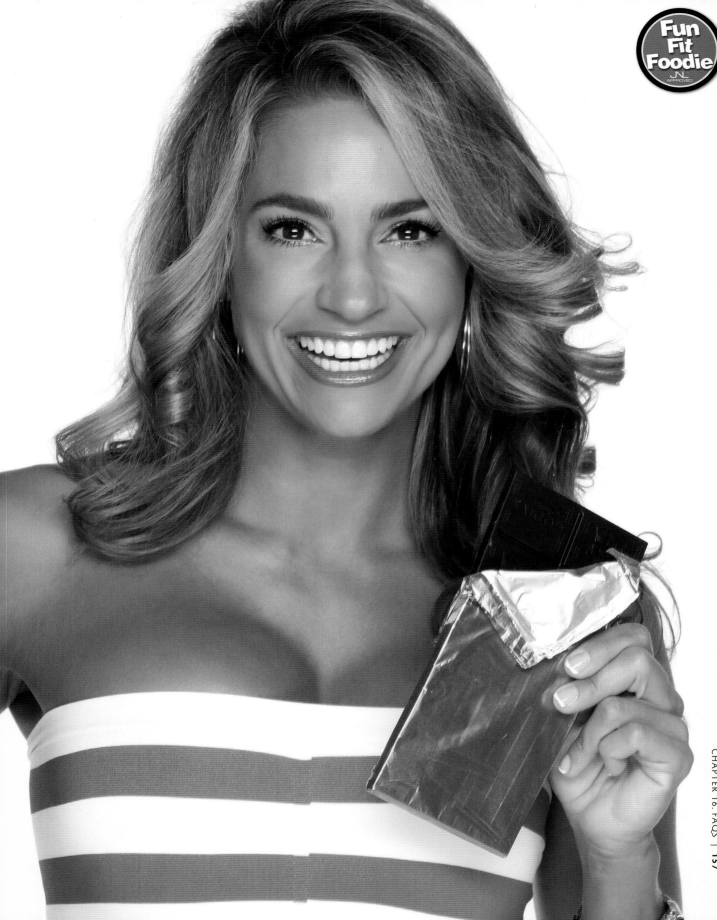

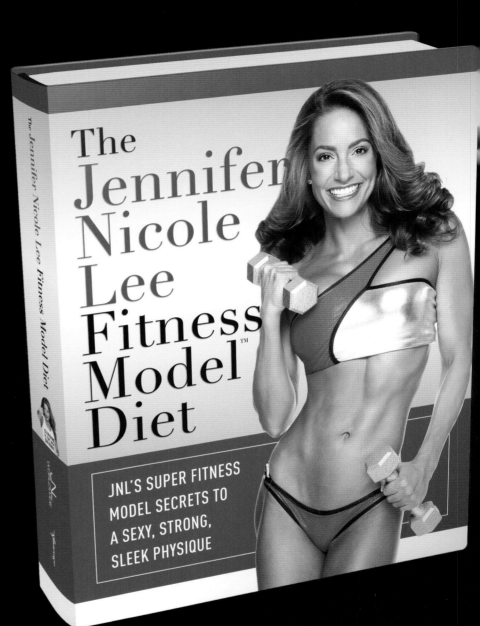

The *Jennifer Nicole Lee Fitness Model Diet*

The
Jennifer
Nicole
Lee
Fitness
Model
Diet™

JNL'S SUPER FITNESS
MODEL SECRETS TO
A SEXY, STRONG,
SLEEK PHYSIQUE

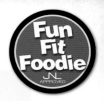

Just to be sure we're clear on this; exercise is more than a choice; it's a key component to the *Fun, Fit Foodie* lifestyle. In my best-selling book, *The Jennifer Nicole Lee Fitness Model Diet: JNL's Super Fitness Model Secrets to a Sexy, Strong, Sleek Physique*, I show you, step by step, my JNL-Approved workouts. You've got to check them out!

I'm actually shocked that some of the top-selling diet books state that the choice of whether or not to exercise is up to you, and that it is non-essential to losing weight. What a lie! I even read a top-selling book, authored by a cardiologist no less, who stated that exercise isn't a necessary part of cardiovascular wellness and physical fitness. Where did he get his degree?

Medical research has established beyond any argument that all forms of exercise, whether it is a brisk walk or a super-duper power pump session in the gym, are beneficial to the cardiovascular system and for the entire body. I am telling you that you MUST treat exercise in this program like an important business meeting with your body that you cannot miss or be late to. Exercise is just "one of the sequence of numbers" that will help you crack the code of healthy weight loss and maintenance. There will be no code-pendency on group meetings, no weekly gatherings, and you won't have to buy "my pre-made and pre-processed" food. Furthermore, you will not have to slave away in your kitchen finely shredding orange peel & peeling/deseeding/slicing papaya for your next "Chicken Raspberry Spinach Salad." This is definitely not the case with the *Fun, Fit Foodie Lifestyle Cookbook!* My book is for the everyday busy person who multi-tasks, and now with my codes to fitness program, you'll be able to get maximum results with small but smart amounts of effort! You will see maximum results in minimum time.

After reading this fit-lifestyle guide you will:

- Know how to increase your metabolism with my simple tips and tools.

- Understand the 3 F's that equal an A+ in weight training.

- Exercise smarter, not harder!

- Understand why weight training is an underestimated lifesaver.

- Know my favorite fundamental weight-training exercises.

- Learn the difference between good and bad carbs and fats.

- Learn why exercising in the morning is the best choice.

- Understand that fitness must start in your mind.

- Learn how fiber is your best friend when it comes to weight loss.

- Learn how not to get bored or discouraged when hitting a plateau.

- Break through mental and physical barriers that keep you from achieving your goals.

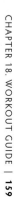

JNL FUSION

THE BENEFITS OF CIRCUIT TRAINING: BLAST THROUGH THOSE PLATEAUS

Let's face it: Plateaus can happen. It is important to remember that if you have faithfully established healthy food and exercise habits as a part of your lifestyle, your fitness goals can and will be attained.

Still, it is important to add circuit training in combination with strength training to reach your weight-loss and fitness potential. This will add an entirely new dimension to your current fitness program. Circuit training allows you to keep your body guessing by adding cardio sprints intertwined with strength/weight training moves. For more information visit ww.JNLFusion.com

TRAINING VERSUS OVERTRAINING

- A successful weightlifting regimen is based on the notion that, in order to build muscle and increase strength, it is necessary to progressively raise your resistance, or overload.

- Muscles must be given adequate time to recover and rebuild so that new muscle can form.

- Progressive resistance, or overloading, can be done simply by doing more reps on a set with the same weight. Also, in addition to adding more weight in your reps, you can add progressive resistance by decreasing the time you rest between sets.

- It is important to never get too comfortable. In order to make great gains towards building muscle you must strive to do more. Your training sessions should get harder and more intense.

- However, when you make your workouts more intense and harder, it is very important that you get enough rest between workouts, and allow enough recovery time for your muscles.

- If this does not occur, you will end up overtraining your muscles. Your overworked muscles will not get bigger, but will instead get smaller and weaker. Your muscles could be easily torn, or permanently damaged, without proper recovery time.

- When training intensely, it's very important to take time off from your workouts. You should consider taking a week to 10 days off every 4 to 8 weeks to keep your mind and body fresh.

REST!

No, I am not telling you to take a 5-hour relaxation session! But what I am emphasizing here is that "Rome was not built in a day."

Don't be like a flash in a pan with your exercise and food plan. Instead, it is best to function like a fire that gets stronger with every twig and branch that is put on top of it. Fitness is NOT an event, but a process. Sure, we all will have "off" days, but we must not lose track of our objective. Keep your eyes on the prize, and aim to attain it slowly! Allow yourself a break.

I have seen it too many times in the fitness industry: people come in with a lot of drive and heat, but they soon fizzle out. Pace yourself. Allow yourself a break. Do not train more than 6 days a week. I don't train more than 4 days a week and people look at me in amazement when they hear this. It is because I have "Cracked the Code" on my metabolism, which has allowed me to have less time in the gym and more time with my family, friends and career. It has given me a quality of life that is limitless! I am not a slave to my exercise and food plan. Rather, they are obedient to me and I have the upper hand, allowing me to burn more calories efficiently and effectively, because I train and eat smarter, NOT HARDER. Give yourself the gift of time to keep your eye on the prize; allow your body downtime to heal, and regenerate the muscle tissue that you are working to grow.

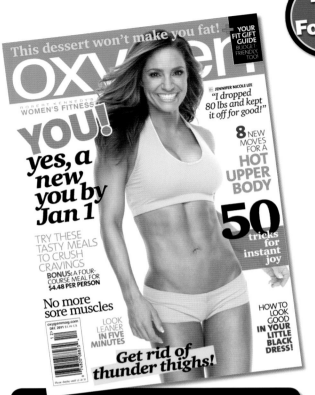

If you loved JNL's *Fun, Fit Foodie Cookbook*, then you will adore her *Fitness Model Diet* book! If you have the goal to dial down your weight, and blast more fat, then make sure you visit www.JNLBooks.com

If you want to train like Jennifer Nicole Lee, and to learn more about the JNL FUSION method, please visit www.**JNLFUSION**.com

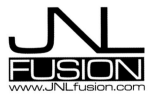

BONUS CHAPTER!

Diet Diva

DIG IN & GET THIN!

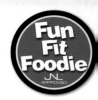

The Fun, Fit Foodie Jump Start Fat Blasting 7-Day Meal Plan!

Co-authored by the Fun, Fit Foodie Jennifer Nicole Lee & "The Diet Diva" Unni Greene

Okay foodies, this plan is for those who need to lose a little bit of weight and really want to rev up their fat burning furnace. It's been designed so you will shed fat pounds while maintaining your sexy, strong, sleek muscle tone. So dig in and get thin!

I thank my dear fitness friend "The Diet Diva" for designing this 7-Day Jump Start for all of us who may need a little more help in shedding some pounds! She is a shining example, as she is a proud mother of four children, and who "claims" she is over 45 years old! She is proof that there are no excuses, and that by fueling your body with the right "super foods" you can and will have the body of your dreams and the energy to match. Enjoy this fabulously fit mother who is over 45 as she shares with us her fat torching and muscle fueling blue print of a meal plan that will help us get rid of those unwanted fat pounds!

Notes: The meals on this plan are all composed of approximately 30% complex carbohydrates, consumed early in the day, 40% protein, and 30% "good" fats and approximately 1,200 calories per day.

FAT BLASTING JUMP START GUIDE LINES:

On this meal plan you should make sure to take a daily multivitamin, as always, stay clear of sugar, sweets and alcohol, and restrict your sodium intake as well as drinking at least 8-10 glasses of water per day.

KEEP YOUR EYE ON THE PRIZE! On this plan, you need to stay consistent. Stick to the plan. There is not a lot of variety but you will boost your metabolic rate significantly. Stick to the timing, as well. You must eat every three hours, starting with breakfast within one hour of waking up.

STICK TO YOUR SCHEDULED MEALS! Your meals are fueling your revved up metabolism. To keep the fire burning you have to fuel it. So eat all of your meals.

STICK TO THE RIGHT FOODS. On this meal plan we are not recommending cruciferous veggies. A short list of cruciferous vegetables are broccoli, brussels sprouts, cauliflower, and bok choy. Your protein sources should be lean and clean.

"PEE OFF THE POUNDS." Sorry to be so frank about it, but when you are reminded to drink water this way, you will remember! It just a saying you will never forget! Make sure you drink as much water as possible. We suggest at least 100 oz per day. That is roughly 5 – 6 medium sized water bottles per day. This will improve your metabolic rate as well. You may become very familiar with the bathroom, but that's a great sign that your metabolism is revving up and you are shedding fat!

NOTE: (Supports a woman weighing 125 lbs or more)

JUMP START 7-DAY MEAL PLAN:

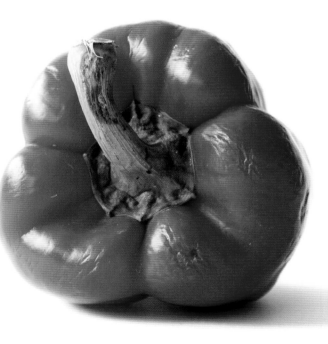

Day One:

BREAKFAST:

- 1 egg, 3 egg whites or ½ cup Egg beater
- ½ cup instant oatmeal mixed with water
- Black coffee or green tea

CALORIES: 233 **FAT:** 9 g **PROTEIN:** 23g **CARBS:** 30g **SODIUM:** 287 mg

SNACK:

- Your JNL Fusion Protein shake

CALORIES: 160 **FAT:** 2g **PROTEIN:** 23g **CARBS:** 3g **SODIUM:** 150 mg

LUNCH:

- 4 oz skinless chicken breast or fish, grilled or steamed
- ½ cup brown rice
- 1 cup asparagus
- 2 cups green salad
- 1 tbsp low calorie dressing

CALORIES: 333 **FAT:** 5g **PROTEIN:** 30g **CARBS:** 31g **SODIUM:** 229 mg

SNACK:

- Protein shake mixed with water. Mix in blender, add ice (optional)

CALORIES: 160, **FAT:** 2g **PROTEIN:** 23g, **CARBS:** 3g, **SODIUM:** 150 mg

or

- 9 almonds
- 2 cups celery or cucumber

CALORIES: 100 **FAT:** 5g **PROTEIN:** 3g **CARBS:** 5g, **SODIUM:** 150 mg

DINNER:

- 4 oz chicken or turkey no skin, grilled
- 1 cup zucchini
- 1 cup asparagus
- 3 cups mixed salad greens

CALORIES: 260, **FAT:** 2g **PROTEIN:** 36g, **CARBS:** 25 g, **SODIUM:** 120 mg

DAILY CALORIES: 1,246
FAT: 20 -24 g, **PROTEIN:** 135 g, **CARBS:** 92g,
SODIUM: 1,086 mg

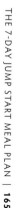

Day Two:

BREAKFAST:

- 1 cup Egg beater
- 1 cup spinach
- 1 toasted whole grain English muffin
- Black coffee or green tea

CALORIES: 267 **FAT:** 3 g **PROTEIN:** 33g **CARBS:** 30g **SODIUM:** 287 mg

SNACK:

- Protein shake mixed with water. Mix in blender, add ice (optional)

CALORIES: 160 **FAT:** 2g **PROTEIN:** 23g **CARBS:** 3g **SODIUM:** 150 mg

LUNCH:

- 4 oz water packed tuna
- ½ whole grain pita pocket
- 1 cup asparagus
- 2 cups green salad
- 1 tbsp low calorie dressing

CALORIES: 314 **FAT:** 5g **PROTEIN:** 43g **CARBS:** 26g **SODIUM:** 229 mg

SNACK:

- Protein shake mixed with water. Mix in blender, add ice (optional)

CALORIES: 160, **FAT:** 2g **PROTEIN:** 23g, **CARBS:** 3g, **SODIUM:** 150 mg

or

- 9 almonds
- 2 cups celery or cucumber

CALORIES: 100 **FAT:** 5g **PROTEIN:** 3g **CARBS:** 5g, **SODIUM:** 150 mg

DINNER:

- 5 oz tilapia, oven baked, or sautéed in 1 tsp olive oil
- 1 cup sliced vegetables, sautéed
- 2 tbs tomato sauce
- 2 cups green salad

CALORIES: 292, **FAT:** 4g **PROTEIN:** 37g, **CARBS:** 30g, **SODIUM:** 120 mg

DAILY CALORIES: 1,212
FAT: 21 g, **PROTEIN:** 135 g, **CARBS:** 99g, **SODIUM** 1,086 mg

Day Three:

BREAKFAST:

- 1 slice whole wheat toast
- 3 slices low sodium turkey
- 2 slices beefsteak tomato
- Black coffee or green tea

CALORIES: 349 **FAT:** 4 g **PROTEIN:** 39g **CARBS:** 39g **SODIUM:** 287 mg

SNACK:

- Protein shake mixed with water. Mix in blender, add ice (optional)

CALORIES: 160 **FAT:** 2g **PROTEIN:** 23g **CARBS:** 3g **SODIUM:** 150 mg

LUNCH:

- 4 oz chicken, grilled
- ½ cup brown rice
- 1 chopped tomato
- 2 cups shredded lettuce
- 1 tbsp low calorie dressing
- 1 tbs salsa

CALORIES:262   **FAT:** 4g **PROTEIN:** 29g **CARBS:** 27.6g **SODIUM:** 229 mg

SNACK:

- Protein shake mixed with water. Mix in blender, add ice (optional)

CALORIES: 160, **FAT:** 2g **PROTEIN:** 23g, **CARBS:** 3g, **SODIUM:** 150 mg

or

- 9 almonds
- 2 cups celery or cucumber

CALORIES: 100 **FAT:** 5g **PROTEIN:** 3g **CARBS:** 5g, **SODIUM:** 150 mg

DINNER:

- 4 oz grilled or baked skinless turkey
- 3 cups salad greens
- 1 tbsp low calorie salad dressing

CALORIES: 260, **FAT:** 2g **PROTEIN:** 36g, **CARBS:** 25 g, **SODIUM:** 120 mg

DAILY CALORIES: 1,146
FAT: 23.3g, **PROTEIN:** 115 g, **CARBS:** 88g,

Day Four:

BREAKFAST:

- 1 egg, 3 egg whites or ½ cup Egg beater
- ½ cup instant oatmeal mixed with water
- Black coffee or green tea

CALORIES: 213 **FAT:** 9g **PROTEIN:** 17g **CARBS:** 33g **SODIUM:** 287 mg

SNACK:

- Protein shake mixed with water. Mix in blender, add ice (optional)

CALORIES: 160 **FAT:** 2g **PROTEIN:** 23g **CARBS:** 3g **SODIUM:** 150 mg

LUNCH:

- 5 oz chicken, grilled
- ½ cup brown rice
- 1 chopped tomato
- 2 cups shredded lettuce
- 1 tbsp low calorie dressing
- 1 tbs salsa

CALORIES: 270 **FAT:** 3g **PROTEIN:** 30g **CARBS:** 33g **SODIUM:** 229 mg

SNACK:

- Protein shake mixed with water. Mix in blender, add ice (optional)

CALORIES: 160 **FAT:** 2g **PROTEIN:** 23g **CARBS:** 3g **SODIUM:** 150 mg

or

- 9 almonds
- 2 cups celery or cucumber

CALORIES: 100 **FAT:** 5g **PROTEIN:** 3g, **CARBS:** 5g, **SODIUM:** 150 mg

DINNER:

- 5 oz tilapia, oven baked, or sautéed in olive oil spray
- 1 cup sliced vegetables sautéed
- 2 tbs tomato sauce
- 2 cups green salad

CALORIES:355, **FAT:** 4g **PROTEIN:** 39g, **CARBS:** 25 g, **SODIUM:** 120 mg

DAILY CALORIES: 1,149
FAT: 22.8g, **PROTEIN:** 108 g, **CARBS:** 92g,

Day Five:

BREAKFAST:

- ½ cup Egg beater
- ½ cup spinach
- 1 toasted whole grain English muffin
- Black coffee or green tea

CALORIES: 267, **FAT:** 2g **PROTEIN:** 33g **CARBS:** 30g **SODIUM:** 287mg

SNACK:

- Protein shake mixed with water. Mix in blender, add ice (optional)

CALORIES: 160 **FAT:** 2g **PROTEIN:** 23g **CARBS:** 3g **SODIUM:** 150 mg

LUNCH:

- 4 oz water packed tuna
- ½ whole grain pita pocket
- 1 cup asparagus
- 2 cups green salad
- 1 tbsp low calorie dressing

CALORIES: 314 **FAT:** 5g **PROTEIN:** 43g **CARBS:** 26g **SODIUM:** 229 mg

SNACK:

- Protein shake mixed with water. Mix in blender, add ice (optional)

CALORIES: 160, **FAT:** 2g **PROTEIN:** 23g, **CARBS:** 3g, **SODIUM:** 150 mg

or

- 9 almonds
- 2 cups celery or cucumber

CALORIES: 100 **FAT:** 5g **PROTEIN:** 3g **CARBS:** 5g, **SODIUM:** 150 mg

DINNER:

- 5 oz chicken, grilled
- 1 cup zucchini
- 1 cup asparagus
- 3 cups mixed salad greens

CALORIES: 292, **FAT:** 4 g, **PROTEIN:** 36g, **CARBS:** 25 g, **SODIUM:** 120 mg

DAILY CALORIES: 1,149
FAT: 22.8g, **PROTEIN:** 108 g, **CARBS:** 92g,

Day Six:

BREAKFAST:

- 1 whole grain frozen waffle
- 1 tbs natural peanut butter
- 1 cup skim milk
- 1 cup cut up papaya

CALORIES: 315, **FAT:** 9.9 g, **PROTEIN:** 15 g, **CARBS:** 45 g, **SODIUM:** 120 mg

SNACK:

- Protein shake mixed with water. Mix in blender, add ice (optional)

CALORIES: 160 **FAT:** 2g **PROTEIN:** 23g **CARBS:** 3g **SODIUM:** 150 mg

LUNCH:

- 5 oz chicken, grilled
- ½ cup brown rice
- 1 chopped tomato
- 2 cups shredded lettuce
- 1 tbsp low calorie dressing
- 1 tbs salsa

CALORIES: 266, **FAT:** 5g **PROTEIN:** 30g, **CARBS:** 31g **SODIUM:** 429 mg

SNACK:

- Protein shake mixed with water. Mix in blender, add ice (optional)

CALORIES: 160 **FAT:** 2g **PROTEIN:** 23g **CARBS:** 3g **SODIUM:** 150 mg

or

- 9 almonds
- 2 cups celery or cucumber

CALORIES: 100 **FAT:** 5g **PROTEIN:** 3g **CARBS:** 5g, **SODIUM:** 150 mg

DINNER:

- 4 oz tilapia, oven baked, or sautéed in olive oil
- 1 cup sliced vegetables sautéed
- 2 tbs tomato sauce
- 2 cups green salad

CALORIES: 260, **FAT:** 2g **PROTEIN:** 36g, **CARBS:** 25 g, **SODIUM:** 120 mg

DAILY CALORIES: 1,149
FAT: 28.2g, **PROTEIN:** 103 g, **CARBS:** 115g,

Day Seven:

BREAKFAST:

- 1 cup Greek yogurt
- 1 cup low sugar high protein granola
- ½ cup egg beaters
- Coffee

CALORIES: 263, **FAT:** 2g **PROTEIN:** 36g, **CARBS:** 20 g, **SODIUM:** 320 mg

SNACK:

- Protein shake mixed with water. Mix in blender, add ice (optional)

CALORIES: 160 **FAT:** 2g **PROTEIN:** 23g **CARBS:** 3g **SODIUM:** 150 mg

LUNCH:

- 1.5 cups low sodium tomato soup
- 1 slice whole wheat toast
- 3 oz low fat cheese, sliced
- 2 large slices tomato
- Lettuce

CALORIES: 341, **FAT:** 6g **PROTEIN:** 31g **CARBS:** 40g, **SODIUM:** 150 mg

SNACK:

- Protein shake mixed with water. Mix in blender, add ice (optional)

CALORIES: 160 **FAT:** 2g **PROTEIN:** 23g **CARBS:** 3g **SODIUM:** 150 mg

or

- 9 almonds
- 2 cups celery or cucumber

CALORIES: 100 **FAT:** 5g **PROTEIN:** 3g **CARBS:** 5g, **SODIUM:** 150 mg

DINNER:

- 4 oz lean beef cut into strips
- 2 cups sliced mixed vegetables
- ½ cup onion
- 1 tbsp olive oil
- ½ cup brown rice

CALORIES: 480 **FAT:** 5g **PROTEIN:** 34g **CARBS:** 28 g, **SODIUM:** 900 mg

DAILY CALORIES: 1,240
FAT: 20.2g, **PROTEIN:** 128 g, **CARBS:** 96g

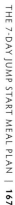

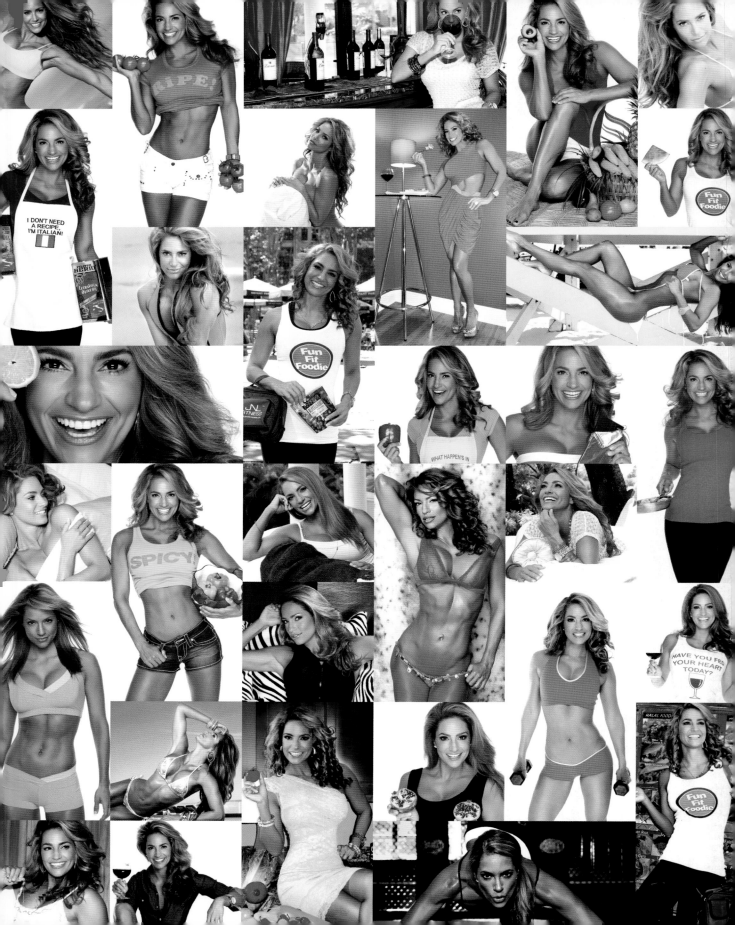

JENNIFER NICOLE LEE is the CEO and visionary power house behind JNL Worldwide, Inc. Due to her wildly successful, globally broadcasted and marketed fitness and wellness products, books, digital products, e-commerce, and merchandise, she is internationally recognized in over 110 different countries. In short, "JNL" is an extremely successful global mega-brand. Mrs. Lee is a fitness celebrity, a bestselling author, a highly sought-after spokesmodel, being the name/face/and body of all of her lifestyle brands, wellness products, exercise equipment, DVDs, home, bath, bedding, spa, and electronic downloads, and websites. However and most importantly, she is a devoted wife and mother, representing the millions of other mom's and wives in the world with a brand they can trust.

"It's my goal and passion to increase the quality of your lifestyle." —JNL

Jennifer is one of the world's most accomplished Super Fitness Models, and is an international celebrity due to her high profile wellness merchandise and key media appearances. Jennifer's career as a top fitness expert and icon began when she lost over 80 lbs after the birth of her children. Her motivational weight loss success story caught the world's attention, after she gained columns of accolades as a professional fitness competitor, holding countless titles and crowns. She gained international notoriety, due to her incredible transformation, and was soon a frequent guest on major national talk shows, such as *The Oprah Winfrey Oprah, E! Entertainment, Fox and Friends, Extra, The Secret Lives of Women*, and most recently being highlighted as the top ultimate "pitch-woman" and presenter on Discovery's *Pitchmen*, showcasing her captivating and strong TV sales power. Jennifer's energy, creativity, and entrepreneurial spirit combined with a burning desire to help others drove her to create the JNL brand. To date she has appeared on a record breaking 47 magazine covers.

Some call JNL the female Donald Trump, due to her uncanny ability to brand, promote, market and sell with the best. Mrs. Lee's passion for business innovation has allowed her to blend lifestyle products and services into the digital realm. Coined as the "Steve Jobs of the fitness industry" she has harnessed the unlimited marketing and sales potential of the internet, creating a plethora of e-commerce sites, and dot coms that rake in a hefty residual income via the world wide web. She is a bestselling author of three hard cover books on diet, nutrition, and exercise, and a contributor to many magazines and ebooks such as *Oxygen, FitnessRx* and Bodybuilding.com. She also runs an international consultation firm, having coached thousands of women from around the world, and has hosted weekend fitness retreats. Jennifer is also a powerful marketing expert, appearing in numerous globally broadcast infomercials for her signature products including the Ab Circle Pro, Mini Circle, and Chest Magic, the Bun & Thigh Wave on top shopping networks, such as The Home Shopping Network. To date, her company and her corporate alliances have three major future lifestyle products soon to be rolling out, with key television media spots secured for advertising. Jennifer is the driving force behind the unprecedented success and future potential of JNL Worldwide. A self-proclaimed "foodie," JNL now shares her passion for healthy gourmet meals that are chock full of antioxidants, made with super foods, with a solid dose of muscle fueling protein, and balanced with fibrous vegetables and "good for you" whole grain carbs.

Want to see JNL in action?

Learn to cook the Fun, Fit Foodie way!

Visit www.TheFunFitFoodie.tv

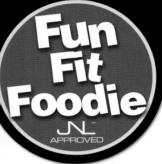

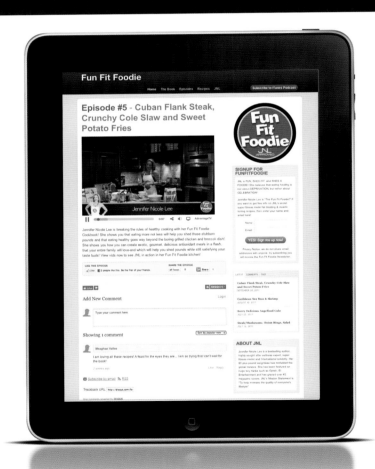

JNL is **FUN, SHE'S FIT,** and **SHE'S A FOODIE!** She believes that eating healthy is not about DEPRIVATION, but rather about CELEBRATION!

Jennifer Nicole Lee is the Fun, Fit Foodie! If you want to get free info on JNL's secret super fitness model fat blasting & muscle toning recipes, visit **www.TheFunFitFoodie.tv** to sign up!

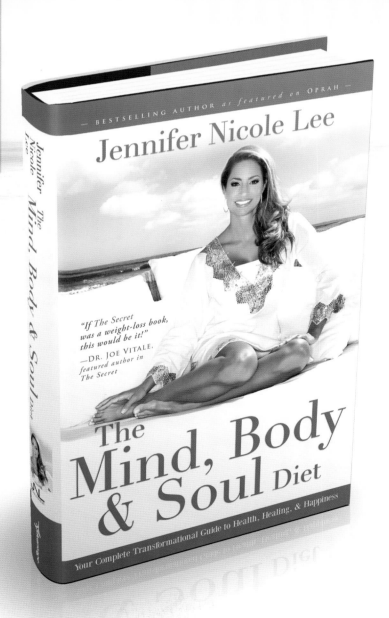
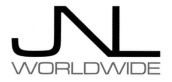

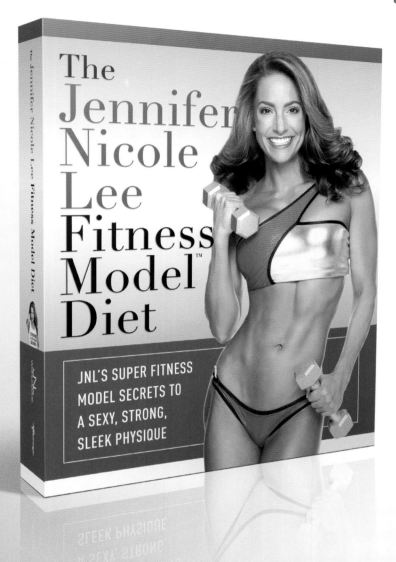
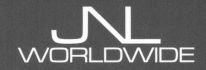